30 Organic Foods for Weight Loss!

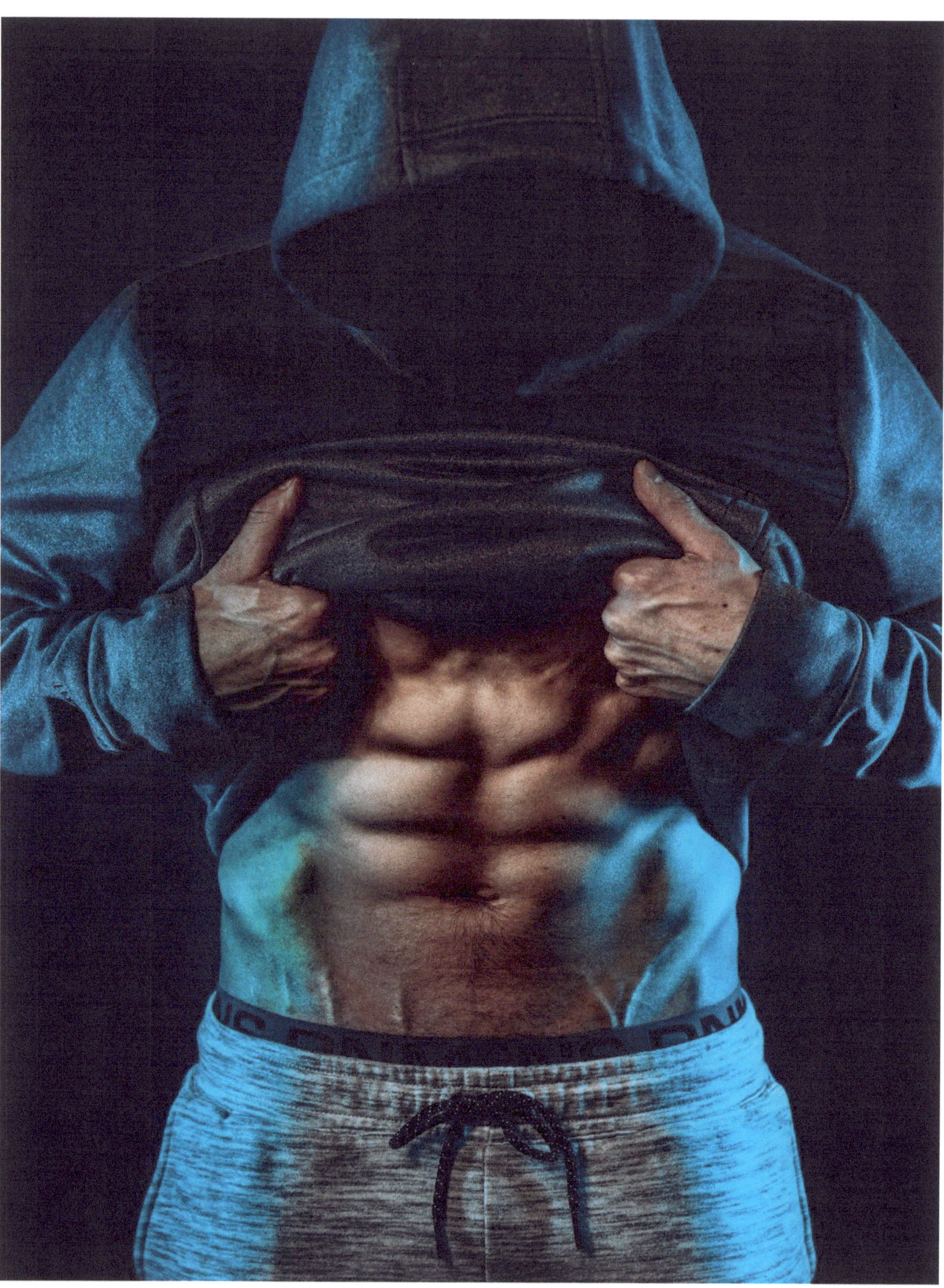

Brief Note :

With regards to deciding ways and reasons for shedding pounds, we wind up gaining either from our friend's insight or counsel from the web.

Be that as it may, on the off chance that you dive further into getting in shape, you wind up observing different negating sentiments concerning the manners in which loads are misfortune.

Truth is told the consequences of each weight losing technique change basically from our day by day supper admission and our body digestion.

So we should hop into the best 10 legends about getting more fit that individuals trust it to work and what doesn't.

Full subtleties are examined in this digital book …

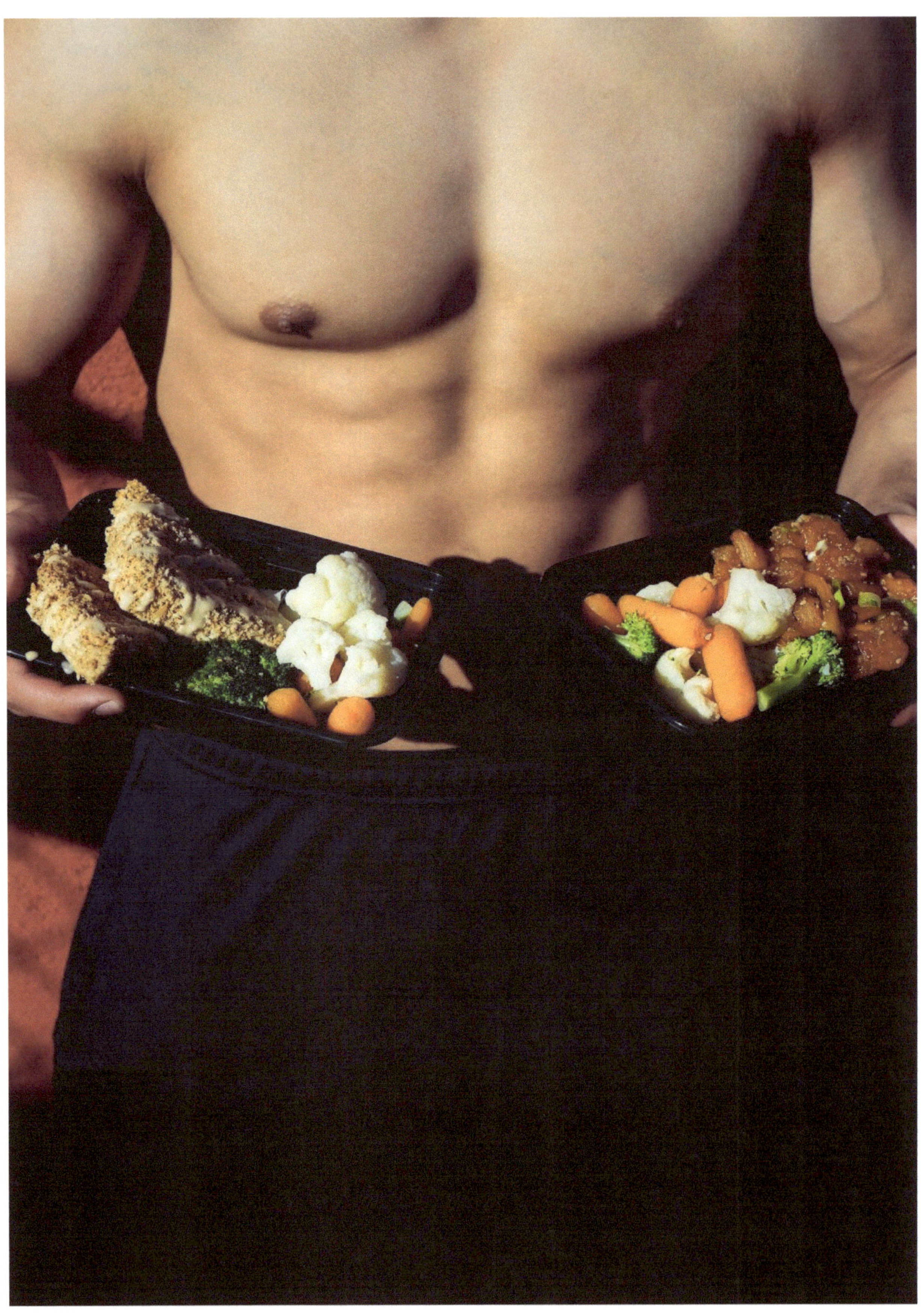

Lawful Notification

The Distributor has strived to be as precise and finish as conceivable in the production of this report, despite the way that he doesn't warrant or speak to whenever that the substance inside is exactly because of the quickly changing nature of the Web.

While the total of what endeavors have been made to check data given in this distribution, the Distributor accepts no accountability for mistakes, oversights, or opposite understanding of the topic thus. Any apparent insults of explicit people, people groups, or associations are unexpected.

In reasonable guidance books, such as whatever else throughout everyday life, there are no assurances of payment made. Perusers are forewarned to answer on their judgment about their conditions to act appropriately.

This book isn't proposed for use as a wellspring of clinical, lawful, business, bookkeeping, or budgetary counsel. All pursuers are instructed to look for administrations regarding skilled experts in clinical, legitimate, business, bookkeeping, and account field.

Table of Contents

1.Fat Burning Basics

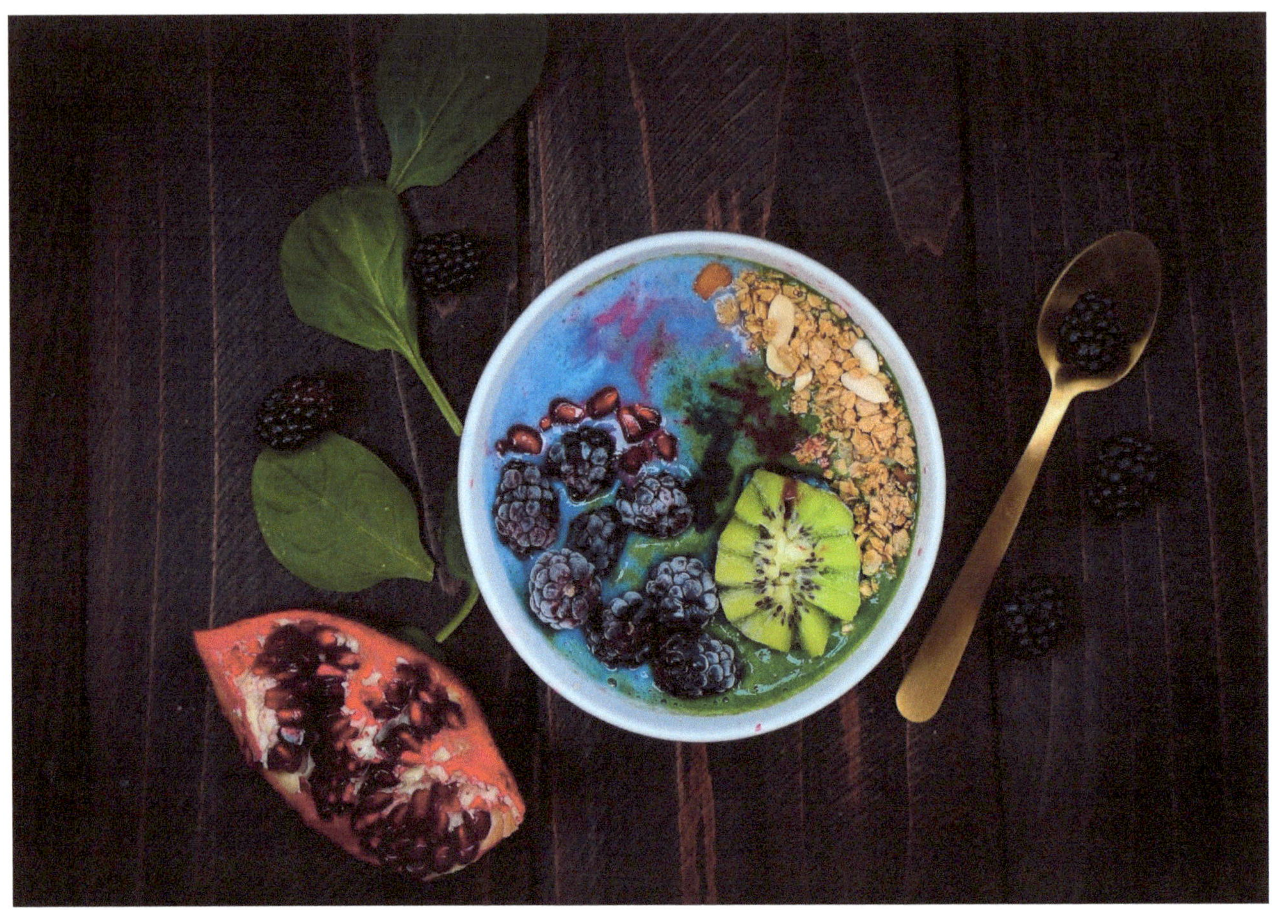

In case you're overweight, you are not an awful individual. You're overweight. Yet, it's essential to lose the additional pounds so you'll look great, feel more advantageous, and build up a feeling of pride and confidence. Whenever you've lost the fat, you'll have to keep up your weight.

In this booklet, you'll find how to shed 10 pounds every month – a pleasant, safe loss of around two or over two pounds per week – effortlessly. You'll feel fulfilled and more vigorous than in the past without feeling denied.
Most Americans pack on those additional pounds by eating some unacceptable things. Changing these helpless dietary patterns is the way to long haul achievement. Information – alongside the correct food – is the key.

At the point when people lived in caverns, they knew nothing about protecting and putting away food. They invested all their waking time and energy chasing and assembling food. At the point when they had it, they ate it down quickly. Rather than putting away food in washrooms or pantries, they put away energy in their bodies as fat to consume during periods when there was nearly nothing or nothing to eat.

Every year, it was indispensable for them to put on a decent layer of fat during the warm run and summer

months. That was the main way they could ensure their endurance during the lean and mean cold weather months.

Furthermore, since ladies bore the youthful, they required more energy to support themselves and their children, and that implied they were normally heavier.

Even though we do not, at this point live in caverns, we have acquired and kept up this fundamental system for fat stockpiling from our chasing and assembling progenitors.

Every last one of us is brought into the world with a specific number of fat cells. The number of these fat cells you have relies upon hereditary qualities. On the off chance that you have a lot of fat cells, perhaps your predecessors were the greatest individuals in the clan, which was something worth being thankful for because they had the best odds of endurance.

You can never dispose of fat cells, yet – sadly – you can add to them. Contingent on what you eat, your body will fabricate new fat cells. Also, similar to those you were brought into the world with, they never disappear.

That doesn't mean you're bound to be fat once you put on additional pounds. It is conceivable to shrivel fat cells. That is the thing that happens when you get in shape. You consume the fat put away in those huge cells. Consider them inflatables. Consuming off the fat inside them has the spare impact as letting the ventilate of an inflatable.

A decent health improvement plan requires a specific measure of admission limitation – the utilization of fewer calories. You consume off the fat by eating less fat and getting more dynamic.

To ensure a lifetime of weight-control achievement, you need to change the sort of nourishments you eat, with the goal that you ingest less fat and still get the nutrients, minerals, minor components, protein, fat, and starches your body needs to flourish.

Amazingly low-calorie diets may assist you with shedding pounds rapidly, yet they'll prompt disappointment over the long haul.

That is because people are hereditarily secured against starvation. During food deficiencies, our bodies hinder our digestion systems and consume less energy so we can remain alive.

A portion of our cerebrum called the nerve center keeps us on an even weight by making a "set point." That is where we feel good. The nerve center decides this point dependent on the fair and square of utilization it's utilized to. It tries to keep our weight consistent, regardless of whether that point is over what it ought to be.

At the point when we radically cut back our food admission, the mind thinks the body is starving, and with an end goal to protect life, it eases back the digestion. Before long the pounds quite fell off. Therefore, we become ravenous and awkward and afterward eat more. And afterward, the eating routine fizzles.

How might you make up for this metabolic lull? The appropriate response is that you need to change the healthful creation of the nourishments you eat. You should eliminate complete calories – that is essential to

weight reduction. More significant, nonetheless, is lessening the level of absolute calories you are getting from fat.

That is how you'll maintain a strategic distance from the starvation alarm in your framework. Simultaneously, you diminish the measure of fat in your food, supplanting it with sheltered, low calorie, supplement rich plant nourishments. This will persuade your cerebrum that your body is getting all the sustenance it requires.

Indeed, you'll have the option to eat more food and feel more fulfilled while burning-through fewer calories and fats.

Plant nourishments separate gradually in your stomach, causing you to feel full more, and they are plentiful in nutrients, minerals, minor components, sugars, and protein for energy and muscle-building. This permits your body to consume off its abundance and put away fat.

2.Fat Consuming Nourishments

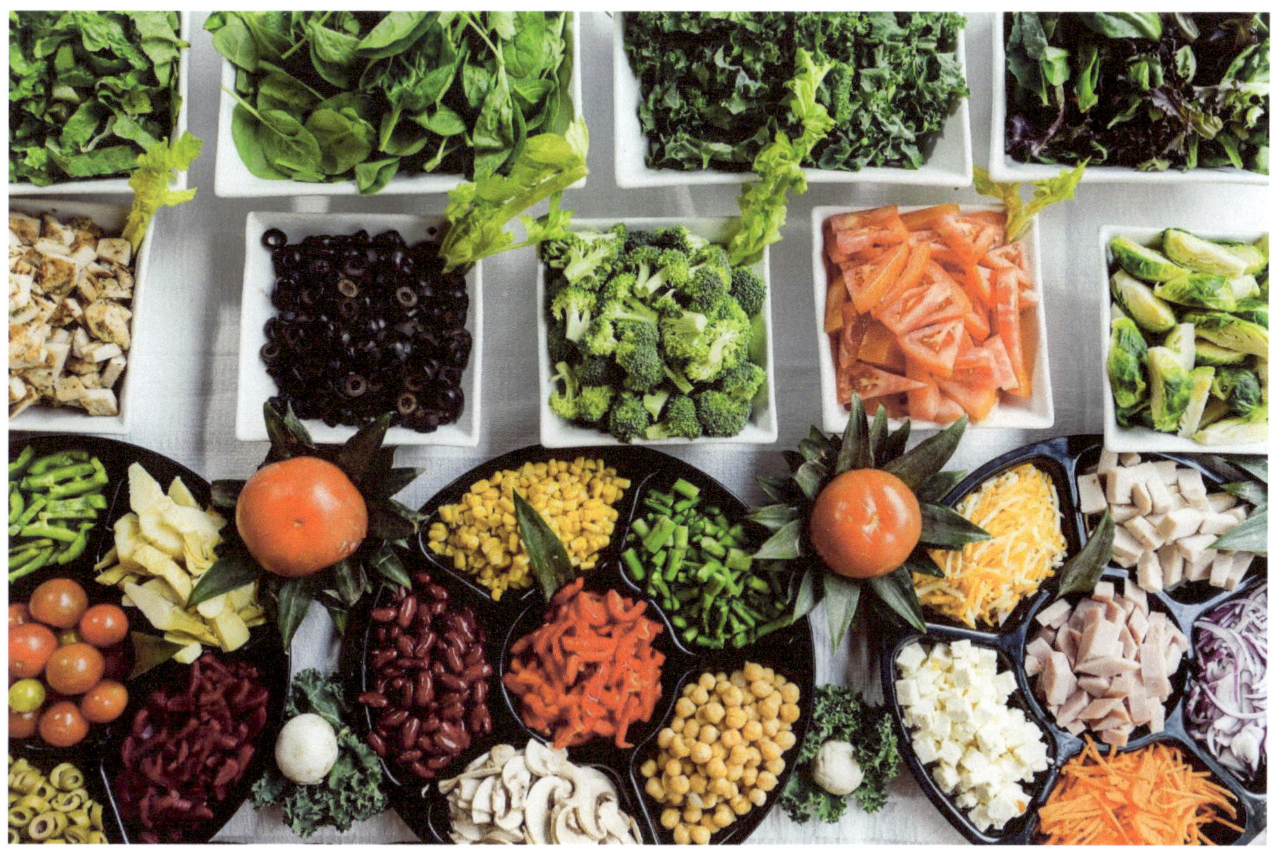

Every last one of the accompanying nourishments is clinically demonstrated to advance weight reduction. These nourishments go a stage past adding no fat to your framework – they have unique properties that add flash to your framework and help your body dissolve away undesirable pounds. These unfathomable nourishments can smother your craving for low-quality nourishment and keep your body running easily with clean fuel and productive energy.

You can remember these nourishments for any reasonable weight-reduction plan. They give your body the extra metabolic discharge that it needs to shave from weight rapidly.

A reasonable weight-reduction plan requires no less than 1,200 calories every day. Be that as it may, Dr. Charles Klein suggests burning-through more than that, on the off chance that you can trust it – 1,500 to 1,800 calories for each day. He says you will even now get in shape viably at that admission level without jeopardizing your well-being.

Yearning is fulfilled all the more totally by filling the stomach. Ounce for ounce, the nourishments recorded beneath achieve that better than any others. Simultaneously, they're wealthy in supplements and have uncommon fat-softening abilities.

Apples

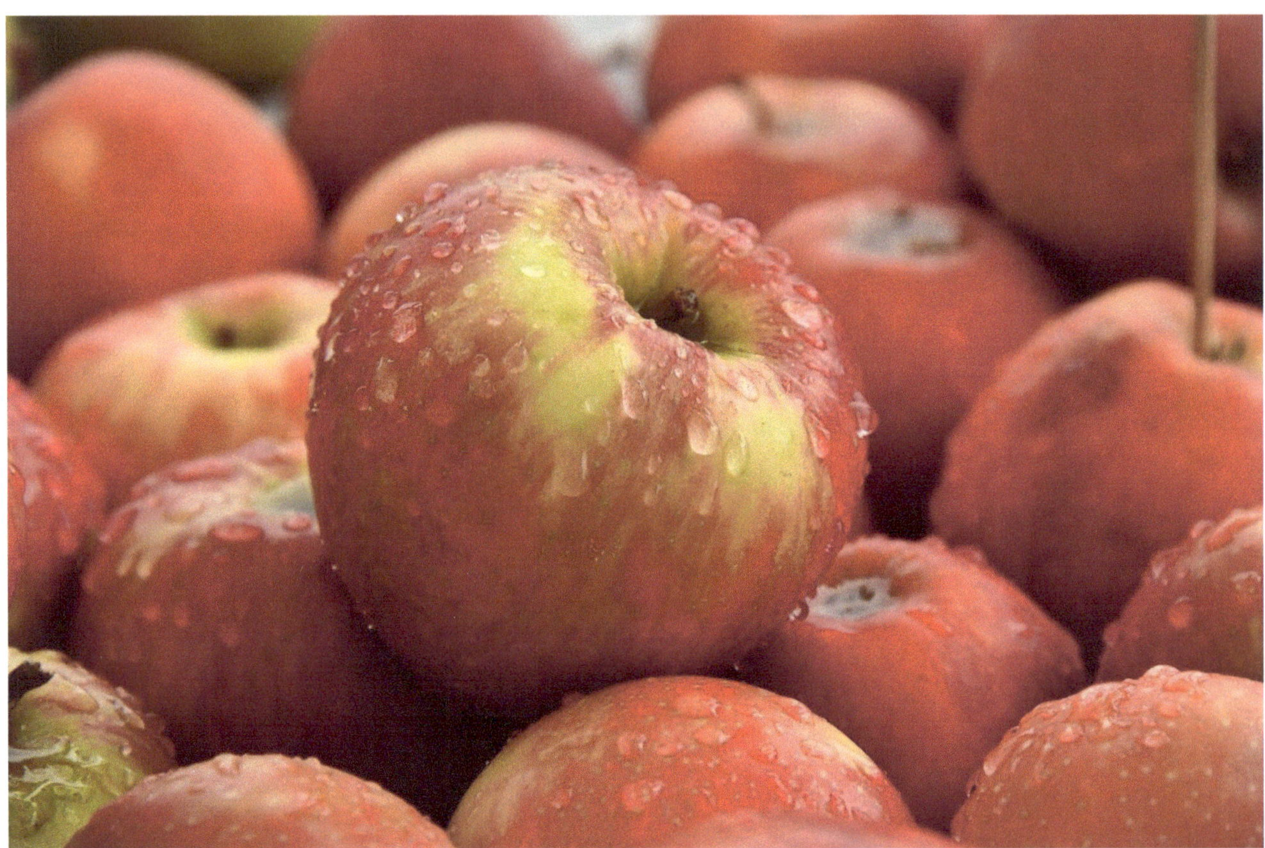

These wonders of nature merit their standing for fending the specialist off when you eat one per day. What's more, presently, it appears, they can assist you with liquefying the fat away, as well.

Above all else, they hoist your blood glucose (sugar) levels in a sheltered, delicate way and keep them up longer than most nourishments. The handy impact of this is to leave you feeling fulfilled longer, state scientists.

Besides, they're perhaps the most extravagant wellspring of dissolvable fiber in the market. This sort of fiber forestalls cravings for food by guarding against perilous swings or drops in your glucose level, says Dr. James Anderson of the College of Kentucky's Institute of Medication.

A normal size apple gives just 81 calories and has no sodium, immersed fat, or cholesterol. You'll likewise get the additional medical advantages of bringing down the degree of cholesterol as of now in your blood just as bringing down your circulatory strain.

Entire Grain Bread

https://59279bou1fppa-fkoe0rn1wzvr.hop.clickbank.net/?tid=1107 2020

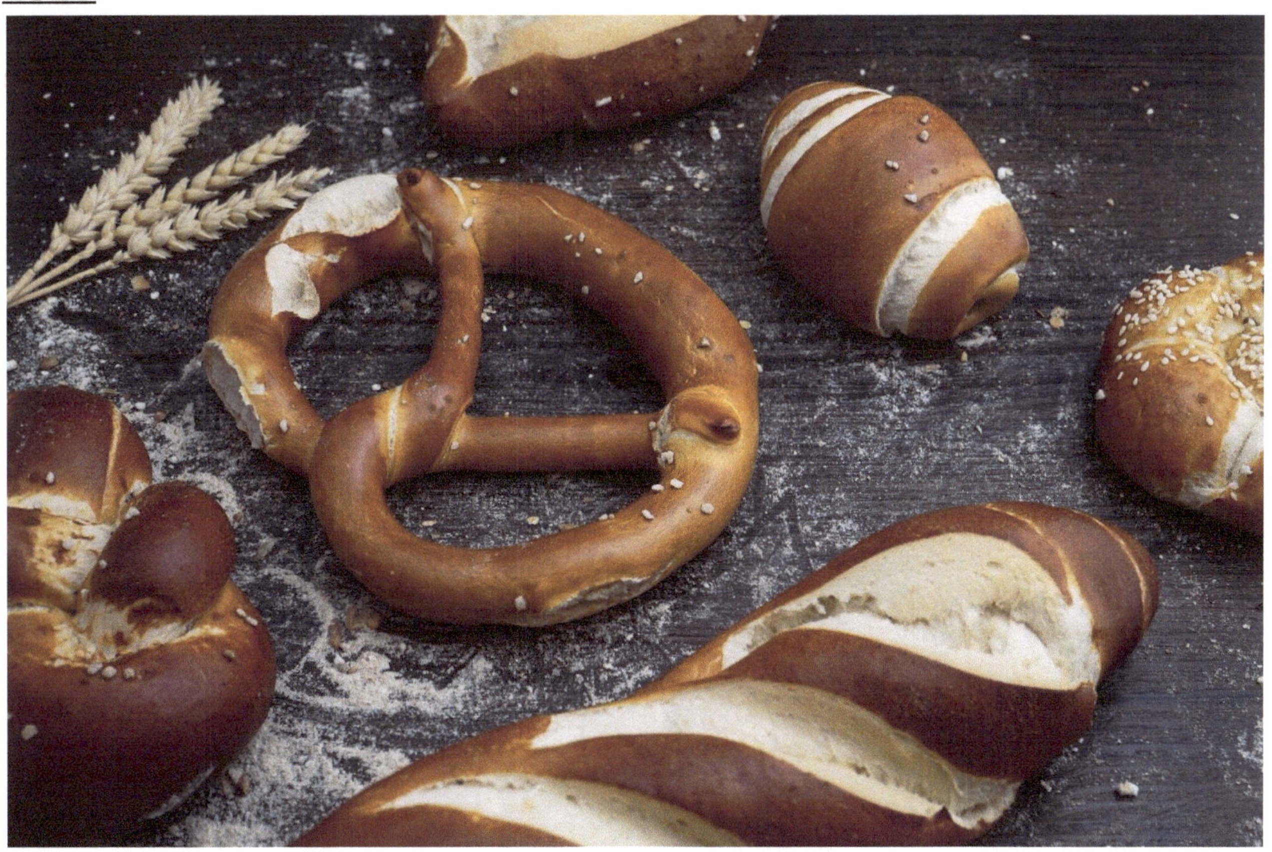

You needn't fear bread. It's the spread, margarine, or cream cheddar you put on it that is swelling, not simply the bread. We'll state this as regularly varying – fat is
stuffing. On the off chance that you don't accept that, consider this – a gram of starch has four calories, a gram of protein four, and a gram of fat nine. So which of these is truly swelling?
Bread, a characteristic wellspring of fiber and complex starches, is alright for eating fewer carbs. Norwegian researcher Dr. Bjarne Jacobsen found that individuals who eat under two cuts of bread day by day weigh around 11 pounds more than the individuals who eat a great deal of bread.

Studies at Michigan State College show a few pieces of bread decrease the craving. Scientists contrasted white bread with dim, high-fiber bread and found that understudies who ate 12 cuts every day of the dim, high-fiber bread felt less craving consistently and shed five pounds in two months. Other people who ate white bread were hungrier, ate all the more swelling nourishments, and lost no weight during this time.

So the key is eating dull, rich, high-fiber loaves of bread, for example, pumpernickel, entire wheat, blended grain, oats, and others. The normal cut of entire grain bread contains just 60 to 70 calories, is wealthy in complex sugars – the best, steadiest fuel you can give your body – and conveys an amazing measure of protein.

Espresso

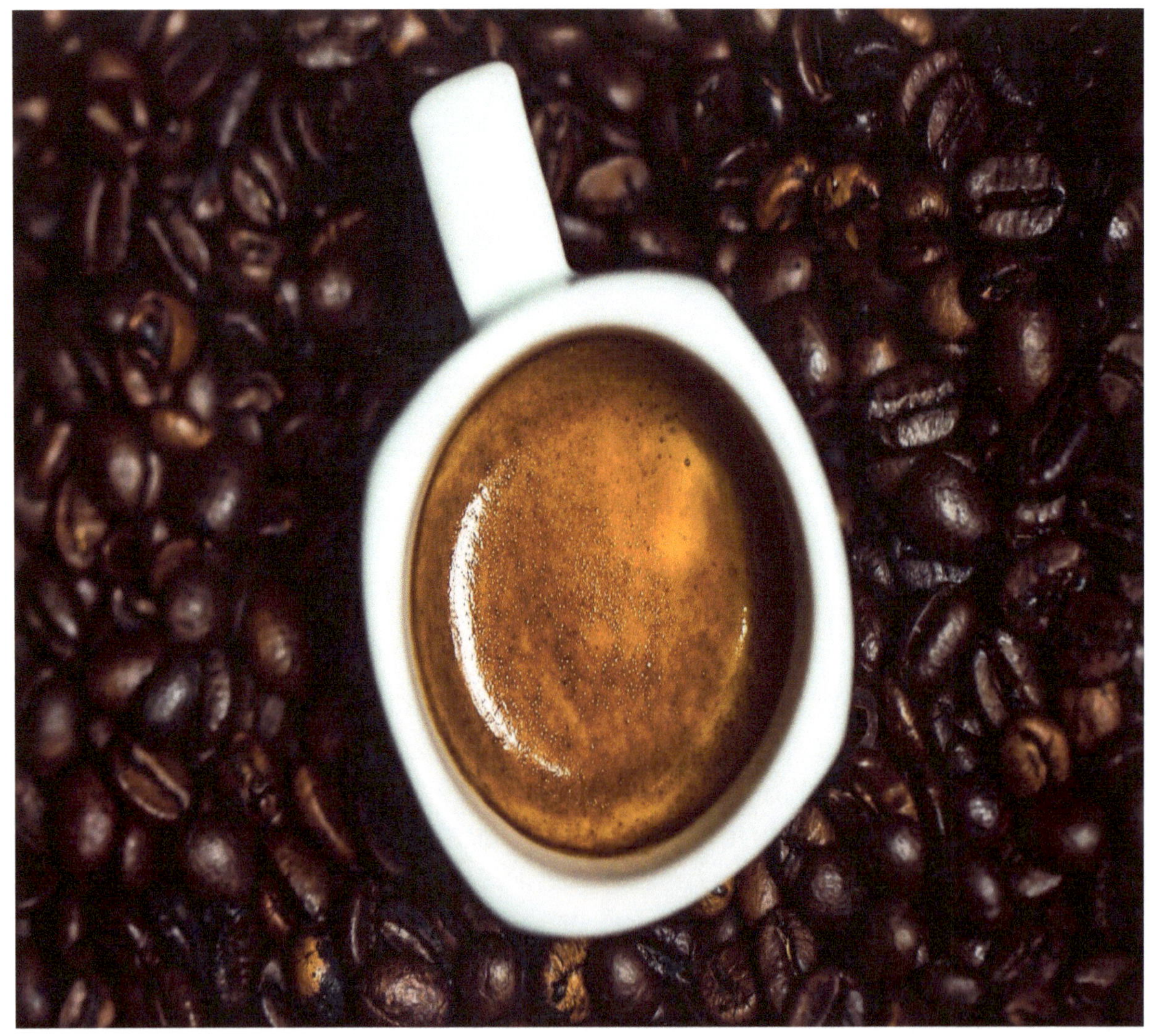

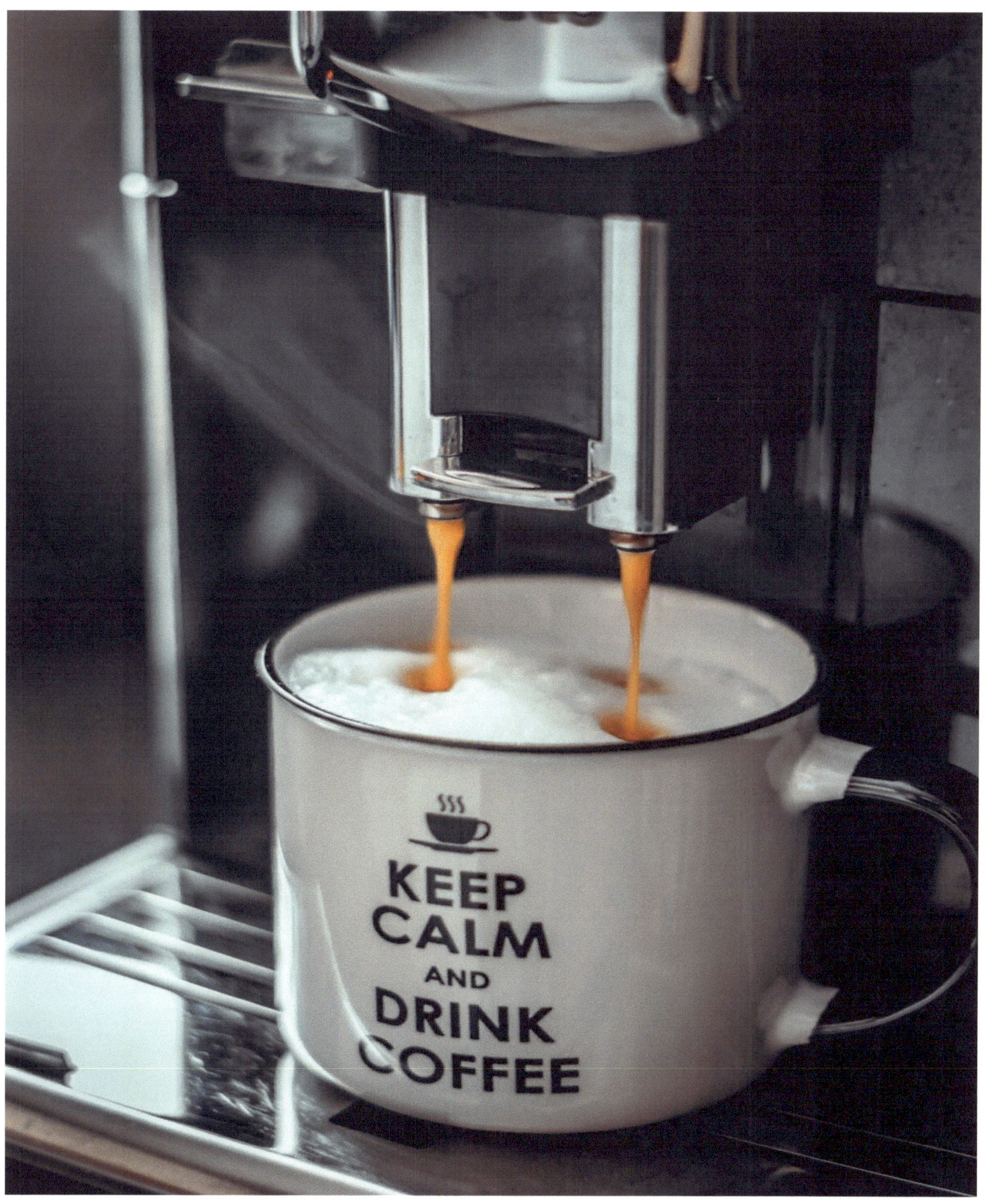
KEEP
CALM
AND
DRINK
COFFEE

Simple does it is the secret word here. We've all caught wind of expected risks of caffeine – including nervousness and a sleeping disorder – so balance is the key.

The caffeine in espresso can accelerate digestion. In dietary circles, it's known as a metabolic enhancer, as per Dr. Judith Harsh of the College of California at Davis.

This bodes well since caffeine is an energizer. Studies show it can assist you with consuming a larger number of calories than typical, maybe up to 10 percent more. For the wellbeing of safety, it's ideal to restrict your admission to a solitary cup in the first part of the day and one in the early evening. Add just skim milk to tit and have a go at managing without sugar – numerous individuals figure out how to adore it that way.

Grapefruit

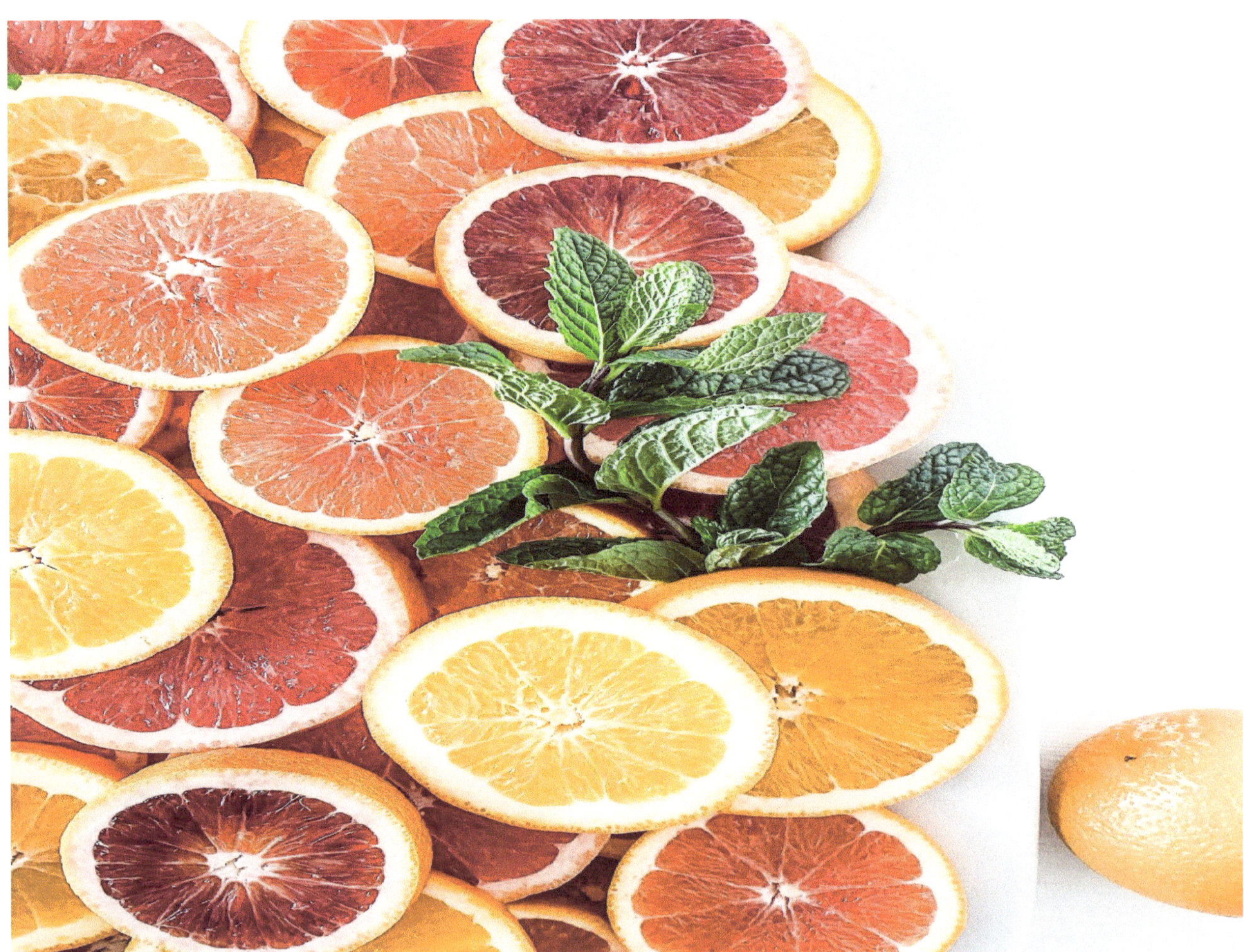

There's a valid justification for this customary eating regimen food to be a standard piece of your eating routine. It assists to break down with fatting and cholesterol, as indicated by Dr. James Cerd of the College of Florida. A normally estimated grapefruit has 74 calories, conveys an astounding 15 grams of gelatin (the uncommon fiber connected to bringing down cholesterol and fat), is high in nutrient C and potassium, and is liberated from fat and sodium.

It's wealthy in normal galacturonic corrosive, which adds to its strength as a fat and cholesterol warrior. The extra advantage here is help with the fight against atherosclerosis (solidifying of the conduits) and the improvement of coronary illness. Take a stab at sprinkling it with cinnamon instead of sugar to remove a portion of the tart taste.

Mustard

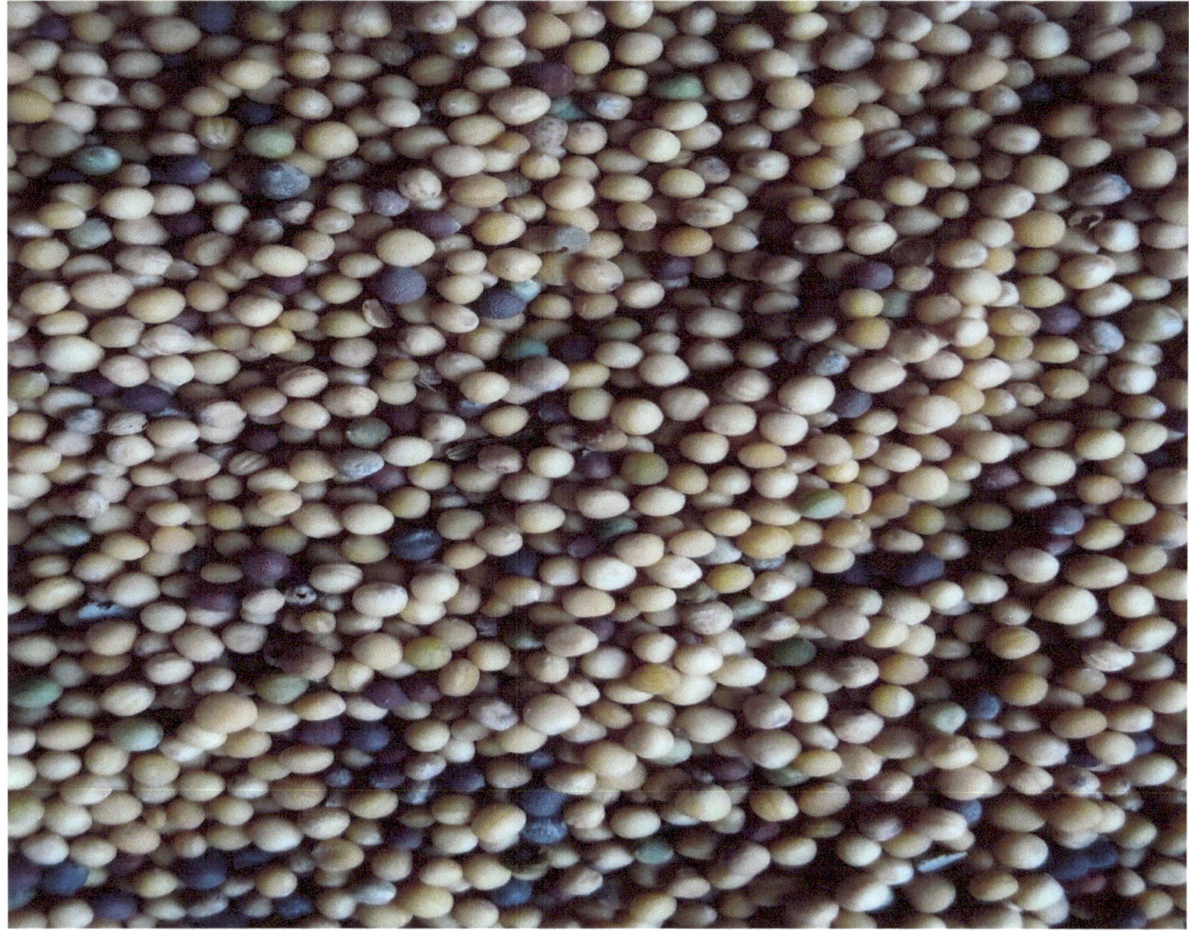

Attempt the hot, hot kind you find in Asian import stores, forte shops, and extraordinary food supplies. Dr. Jaya Henry of Oxford Polytechnic Foundation in Britain discovered that the measure of hot mustard regularly called for in Mexican, Indian and Asian plans, around one teaspoon, incidentally accelerates the digestion, similarly as caffeine and the medication ephedrine do.

"However, mustard is normal and sheltered," Henry says. "It very well may be utilized each day, and it truly works. I was stunned to find it can accelerate the digestion by as much as 20 to 25 percent for a few hours." This can bring about the body consuming an extra 45 calories for each 700 burned-through, Dr. Henry says.

Peppers

https://59279bou1fppa-fkoe0rn1wzvr.hop.clickbank.net/?tid=110 72020

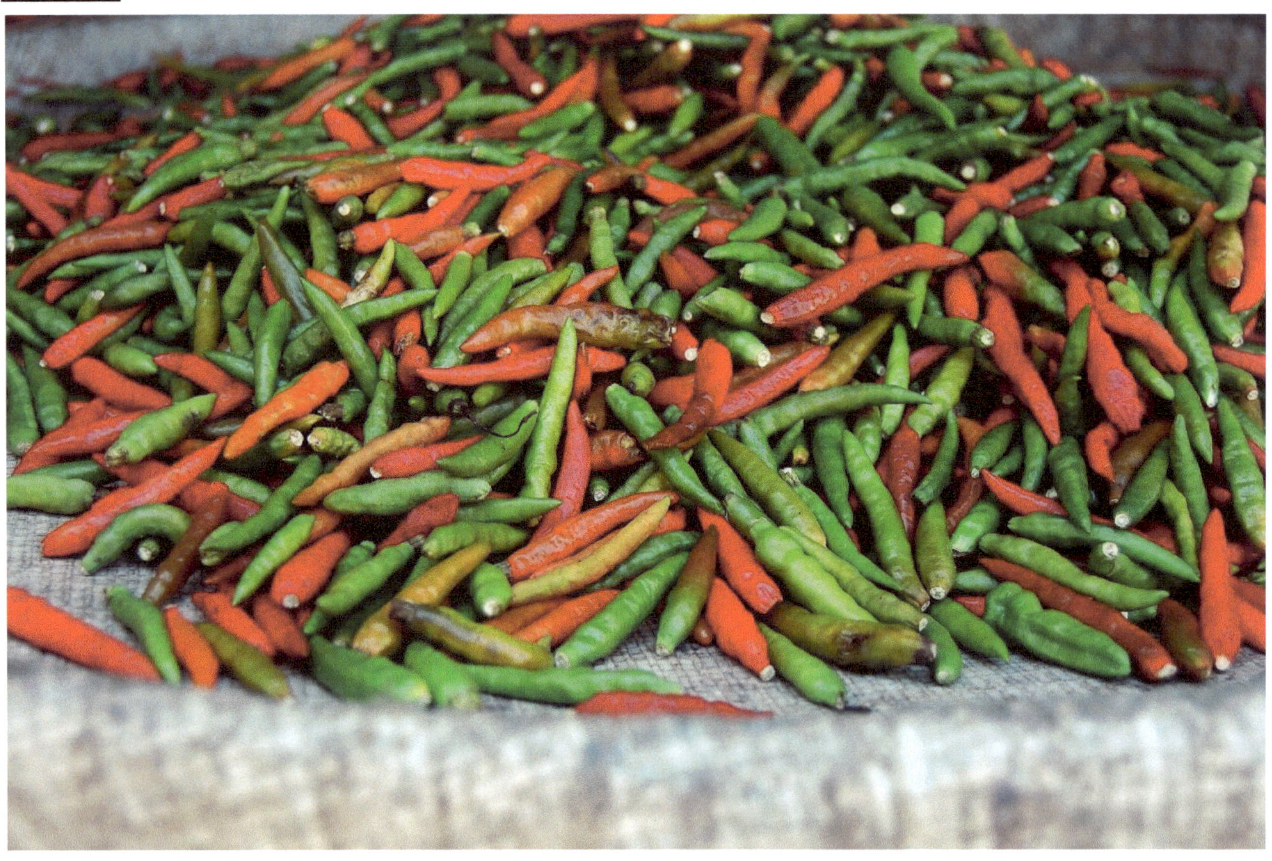

Hot, zesty stew peppers fall into a similar classification as hot mustard, Henry says. He examined them under similar conditions as the mustard and they worked similarly also. A simple three grams of bean stew peppers were added to a supper comprising 766 complete calories. The peppers' digestion raising properties brought about the ideal result, prompting what Henry calls an eating regimen incited thermic impact. It doesn't produce a lot to make the results. Most salsa plans call for four to eight chilies – that is not a ton. Peppers are incredibly plentiful in nutrients An and C, bountiful in calcium, phosphorus, iron, and magnesium, high in fiber, liberated from fat, low in sodium, and have only 24 calories for each cup.

Potatoes

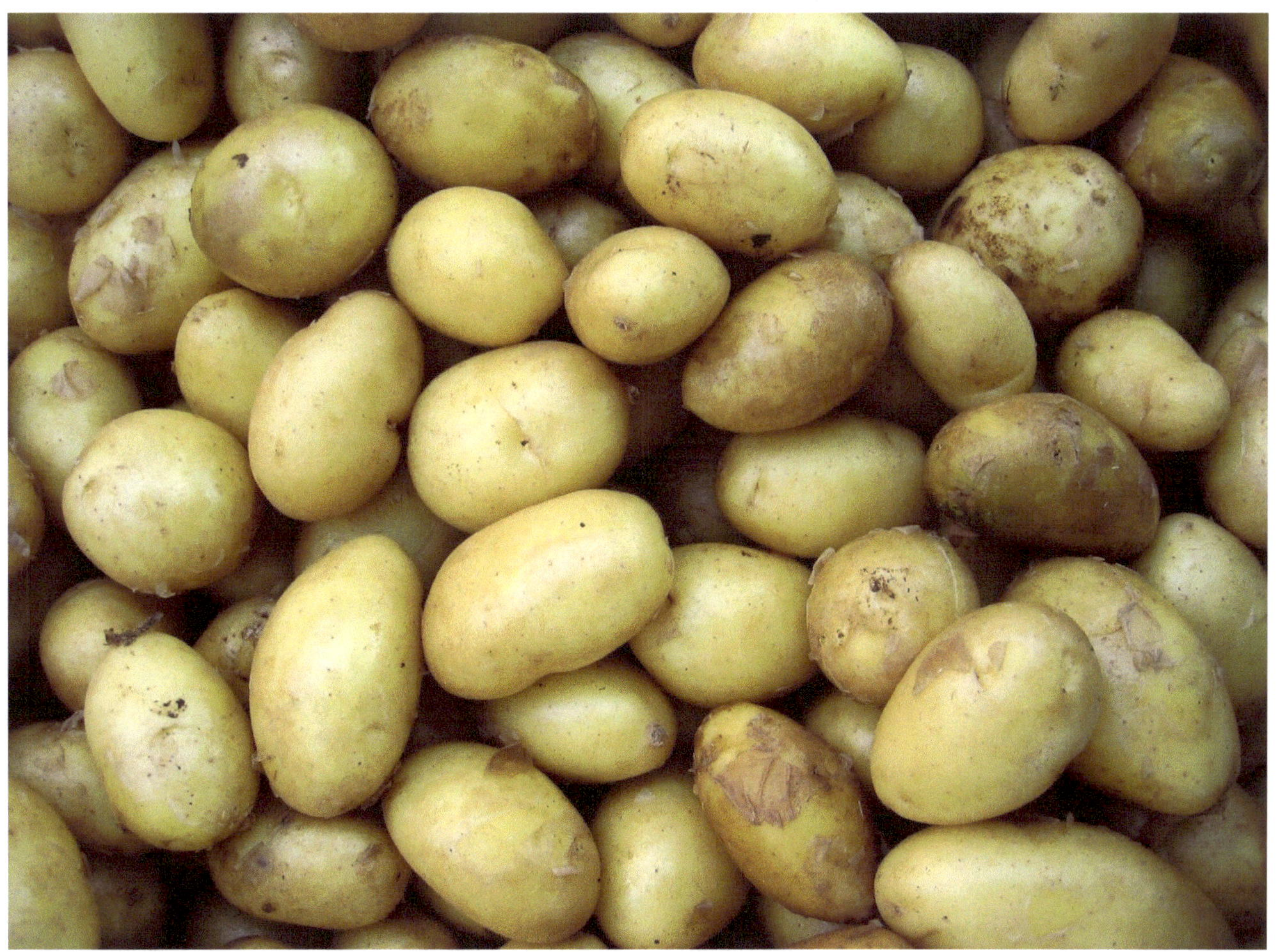

We must have a child, isn't that so? Wrong. Potatoes have built up the equivalent "stuffing" rap as bread, and it's out of line. Dr. John McDougal, head of the dietary medication center at St. Helena Medical clinic in Deer Park, California, says, "A fantastic food with which to accomplish quick weight reduction is the potato, at 0.6 calories per gram or around 85 calories for each potato." An extraordinary wellspring of fiber and potassium, they lower cholesterol and ensure against strokes and coronary illness.

Arrangement and garnishes are essential. Avoid spread, milk, and harsh cream, or you'll blow it. Select yogurt all things being equal.

Rice

https://59279bou1fppa-fkoe0rn1wzvr.hop.clickbank.net/?tid=110
72020

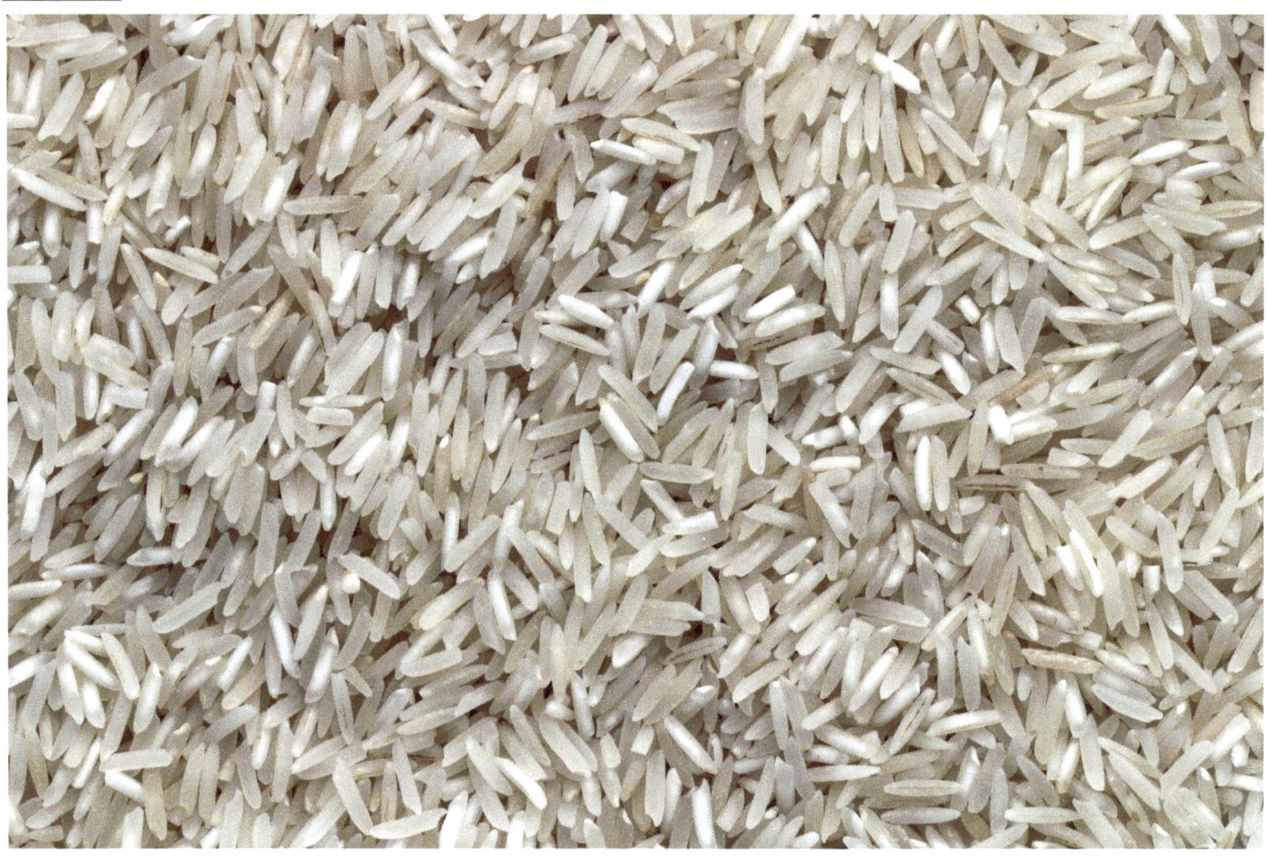

A whole weight-reduction plan, straightforwardly called the Rice Diet, was created by Dr. William Kempner at Duke College in Durham, North Carolina. The eating regimen, dating to the 1930s, makes rice the staple of your food admission. Later on, you progressively blend in different foods grown from the ground.

It produces dazzling weight reduction and clinical outcomes. The eating regimen has appeared to converse and fix kidney afflictions and hypertension.

A cup of cooked rice (150 grams) contains around 178 calories – roughly 33% the number of calories found in a comparable measure of meat or cheddar. Furthermore, recall, entire grain rice is vastly improved for you than white rice.

Soups

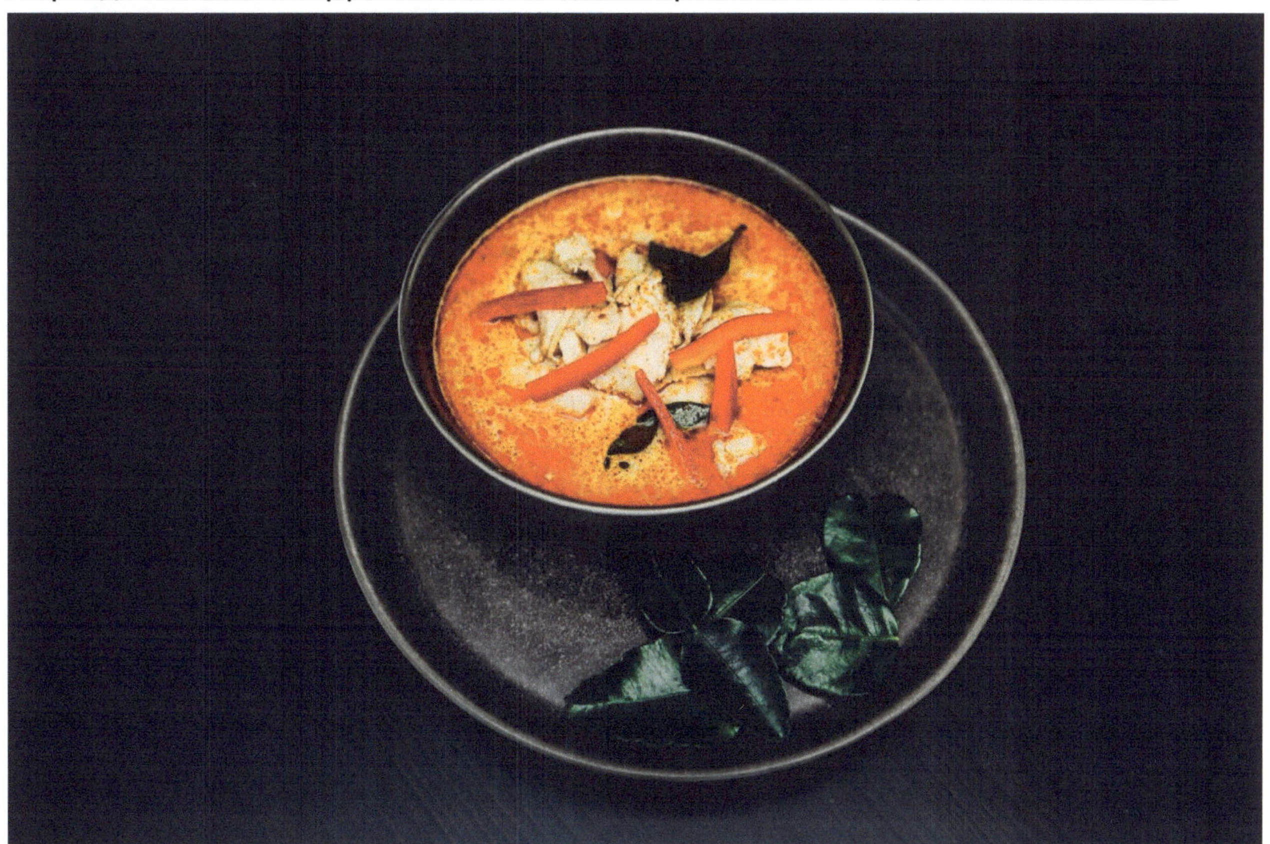

Soup is beneficial for you! Perhaps not the canned assortments from the store – but rather antiquated, custom made soup advances weight reduction. An investigation by Dr. John Foreyt of Baylor School of Medication in Houston, Texas, discovered that calorie counters who ate a bowl of soup before lunch and supper lost more weight than health food nuts who didn't. The more soup they ate, the more weight they lost. Also, soup eaters will in general keep the weight off longer.

Normally, the sort of soup you eat has any kind of effect. Cream soups or those made of meat or pork are not your smartest choices. Be that as it may, here's an extraordinary formula:

Cut three huge onions, three carrots, four stems of celery, one zucchini, and one yellow squash. The spot in a pot. Add three jars of squashed tomatoes, two parcels of low-sodium chicken bouillon, three jars of water, and one cup white wine (discretionary). Add tarragon, basil, oregano, thyme, and garlic powder. Bubble, at that point stew for 60 minutes. Serves six.

Spinach

https://59279bou1fppa-fkoe0rn1wzvr.hop.clickbank.net/?tid=110 72020

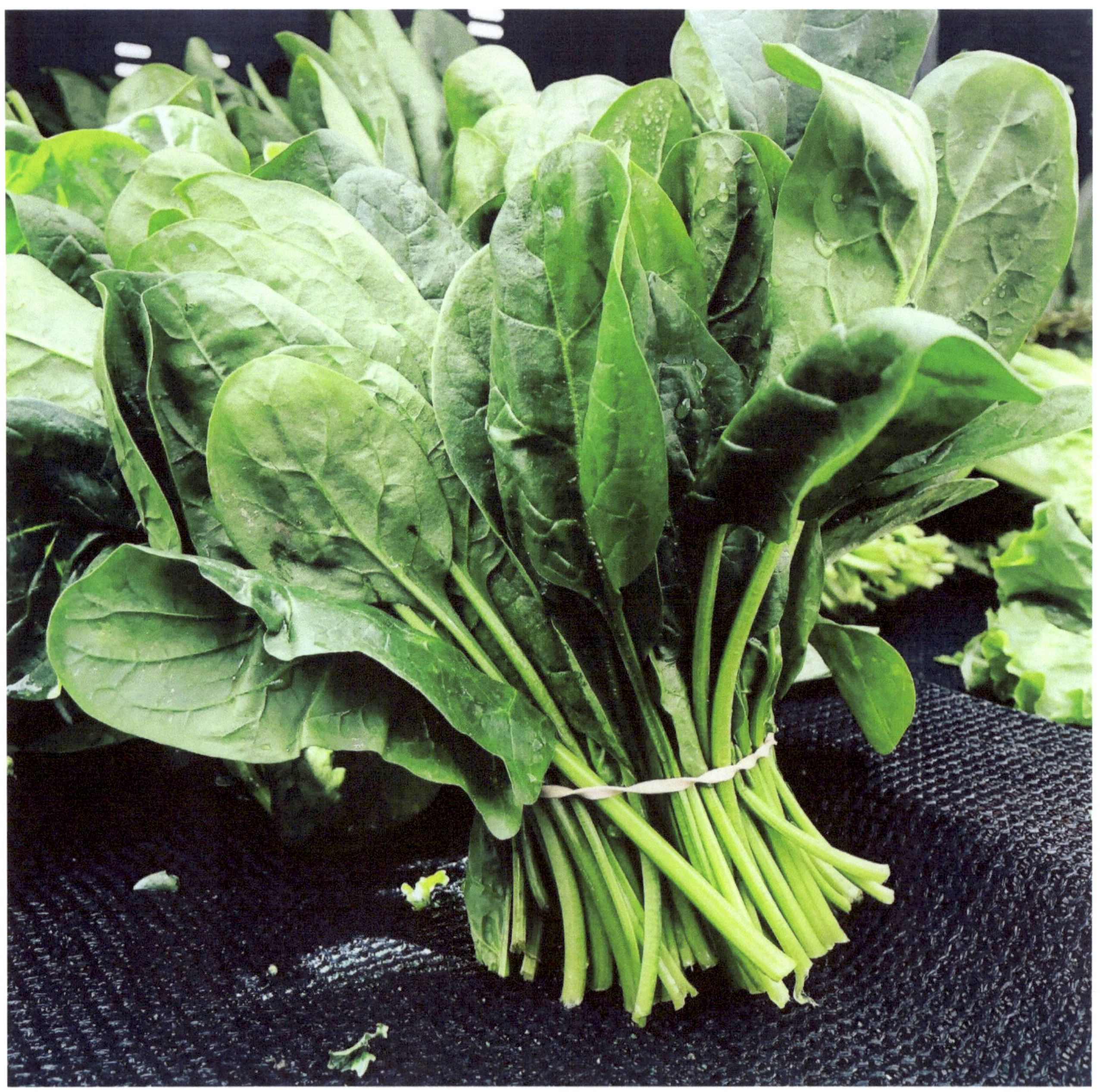

Popeye truly realized what he was looking at, as per Dr. Richard Shekelle, a disease transmission specialist at the College of Texas. Spinach can bring down cholesterol, fire up digestion, and consume with smoldering heat fat.

Plentiful in iron, beta carotene, and nutrients C and E, it supplies a large portion of the supplements you need.

Tofu

https://59279bou1fppa-fkoe0rn1wzvr.hop.clickbank.net/?tid=11072020

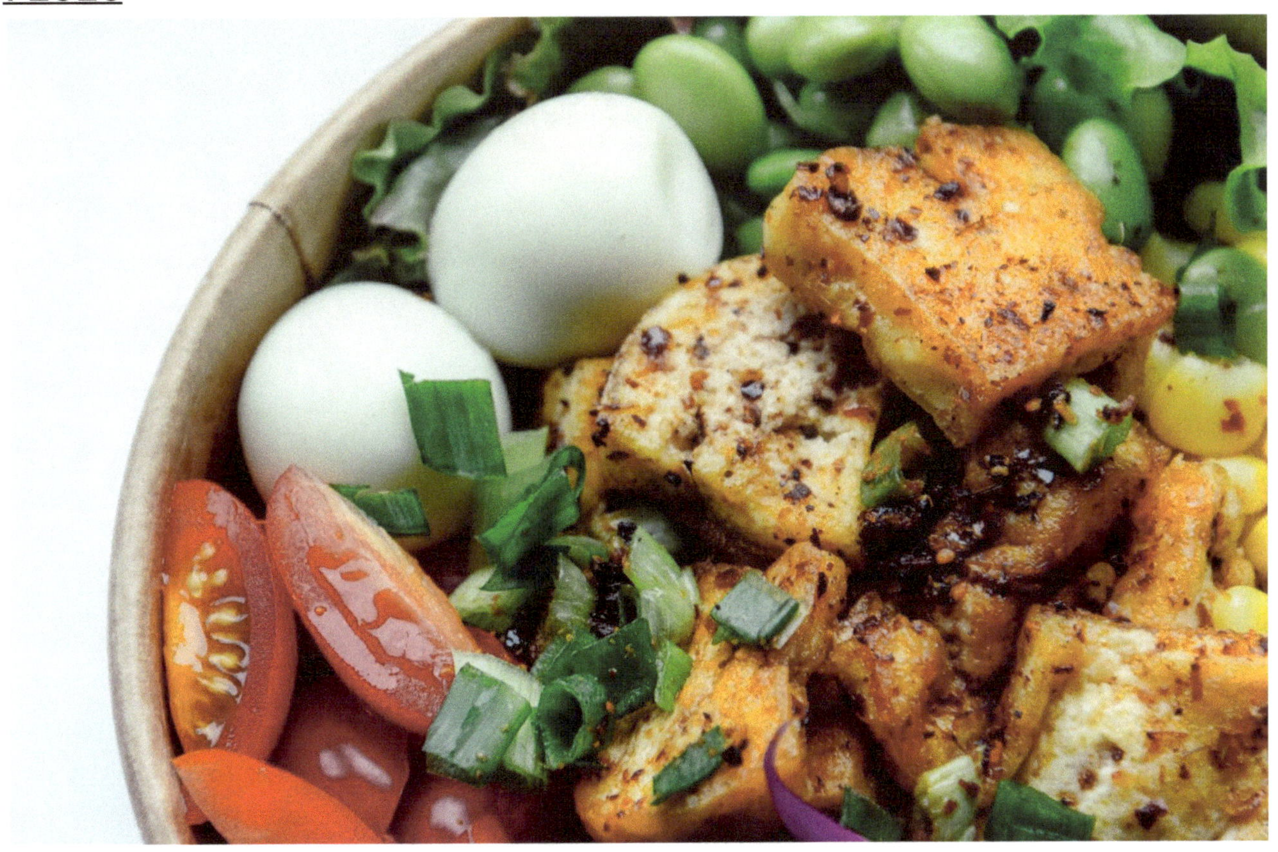

You can't say enough regarding this well-being food from Asia. Additionally called soybean curd, it's essentially dull, so any zest or enhancing you add mixes with it pleasantly. A 2½ " square has 86 calories and nine grams of protein. (Specialists propose an admission of around 40 grams for each day.) Tofu contains calcium and iron, practically no sodium, and no immersed fat. It makes your digestion run on high and even brings down cholesterol. With various assortments accessible, the firmer tofus are goof for pan-searing or adding to soups and sauces while the milder ones are useful for squashing, cleaving, and adding to servings of mixed greens.

3.Powerful Nourishments

https://59279bou1fppa-fkoe0rn1wzvr.hop.clickbank.net/?tid=11072020

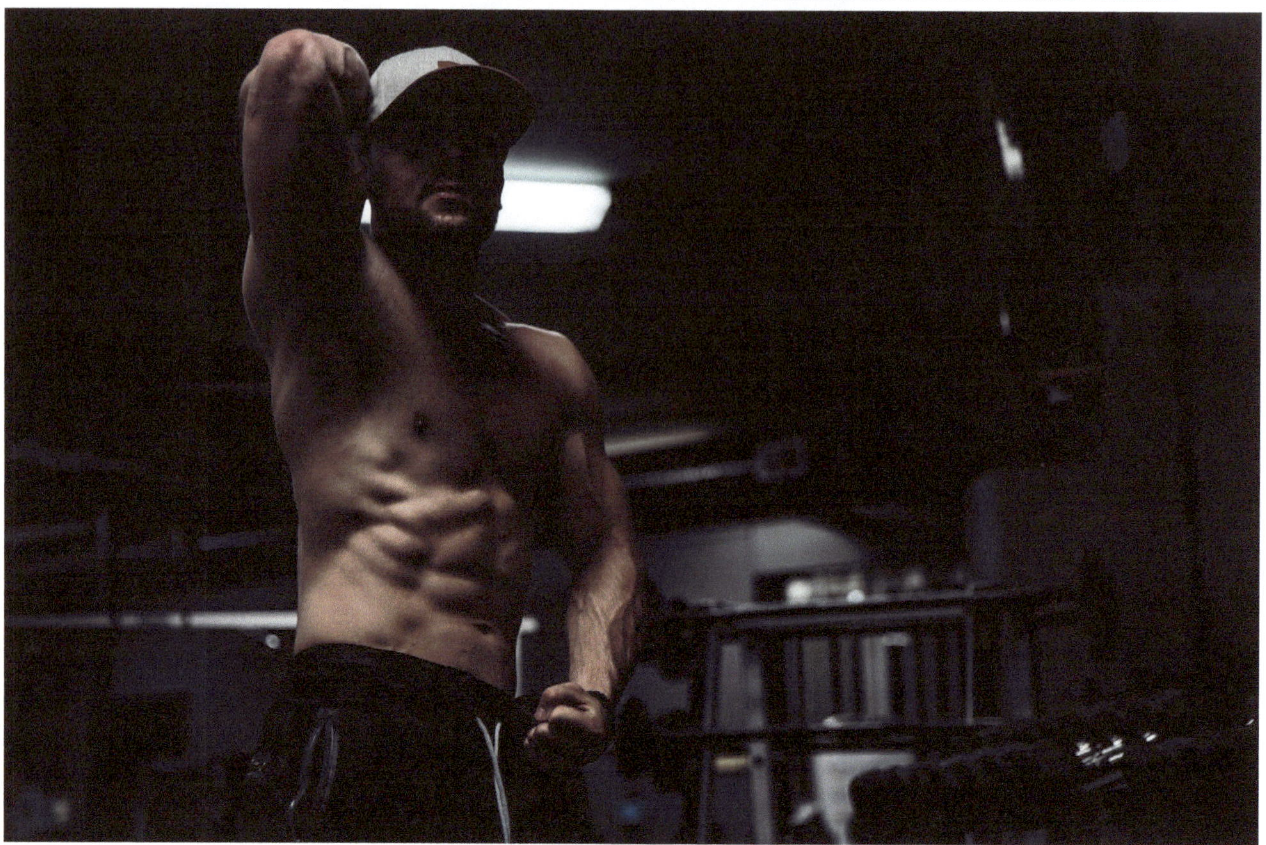

It is unreasonable to figure you could effectively get thinner and appreciate what you're eating with a simple modest bunch of nourishments, regardless of how flavorful, nutritious and fulfilling they might be. So we will add a list of fat-battling nourishments you can eat alongside the incredible food sources referenced in the last area.

They'll loan various tastes and surfaces to each feast and give a wide scope of nutrients, minerals, proteins, and other crucial supplements. Normally, everyone is high in fiber, low in fat, and safe with regards to sodium content, as well.

Many have crunchiness and flavor we've come to want in nibble and snacking nourishments. In case you're similar to a large portion of us, you may have a genuine lousy nourishment nibbling propensity – a propensity you must change to thin down. A large number of the nourishments in this part might be commendable substitutes.

Grains

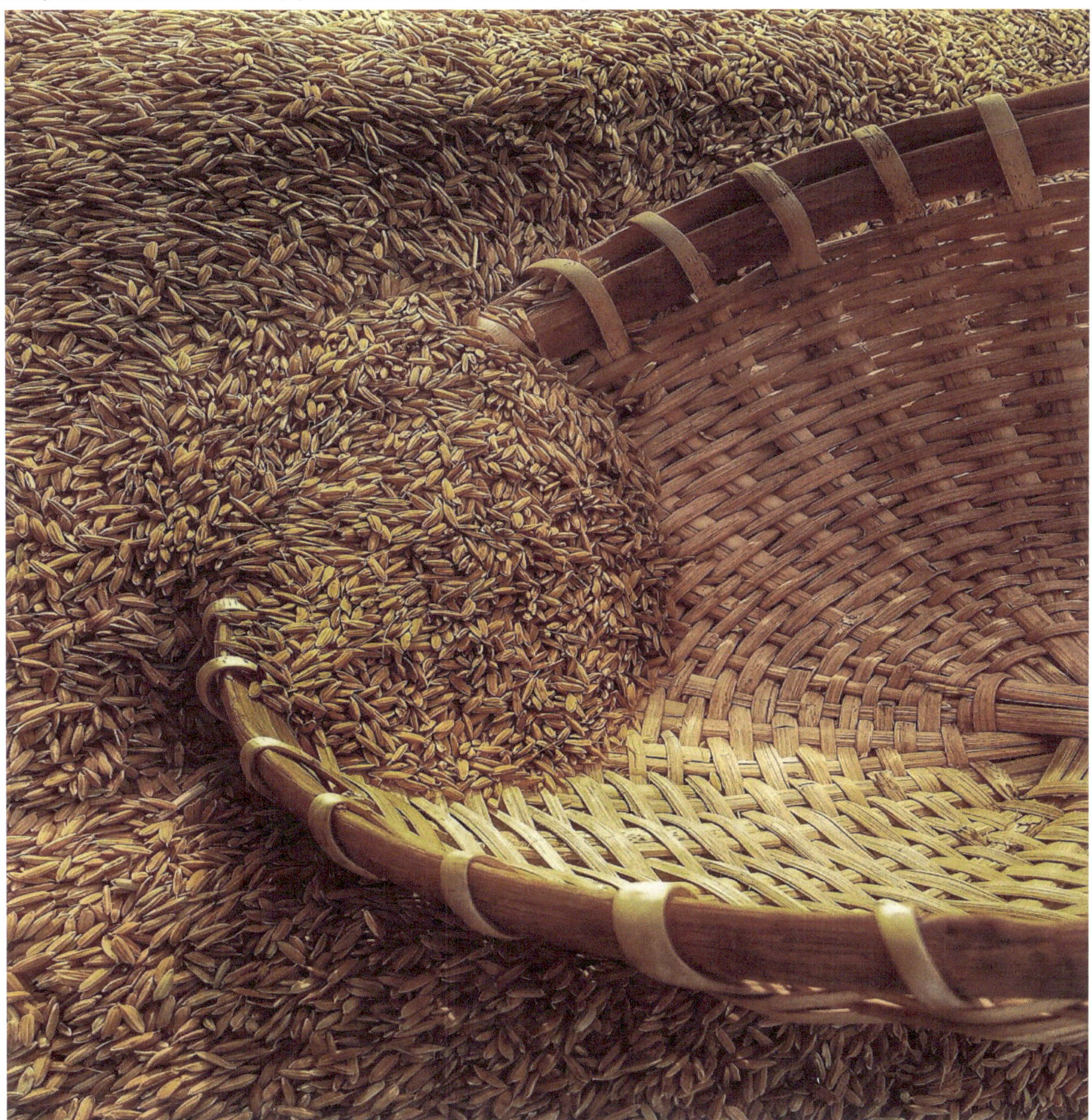

This topping grain stacks off well to rice and potatoes. It has 170 calories for every cooked cup, decent degrees of protein and fiber, and moderately low fat. Roman fighters ate this grain routinely for quality and griped when they needed to eat meat.

Studies at the College of Wisconsin show that grain viably brings cholesterol by up down to 15 percent and has an amazing enemy of malignancy specialists. Israeli researchers state it fixes stoppage better than diuretics - and that can advance weight reduction, as well.

Use it as a substitute for rice in plates of mixed greens, pilaf, or stuffing, or add to soups and stews. You can likewise blend it in with rice for an intriguing surface. Ground into flour, it makes brilliant slices of bread and biscuits.

Beans

https://18c10dji3polfumgzz4x6xcj0n.hop.clickbank.net/

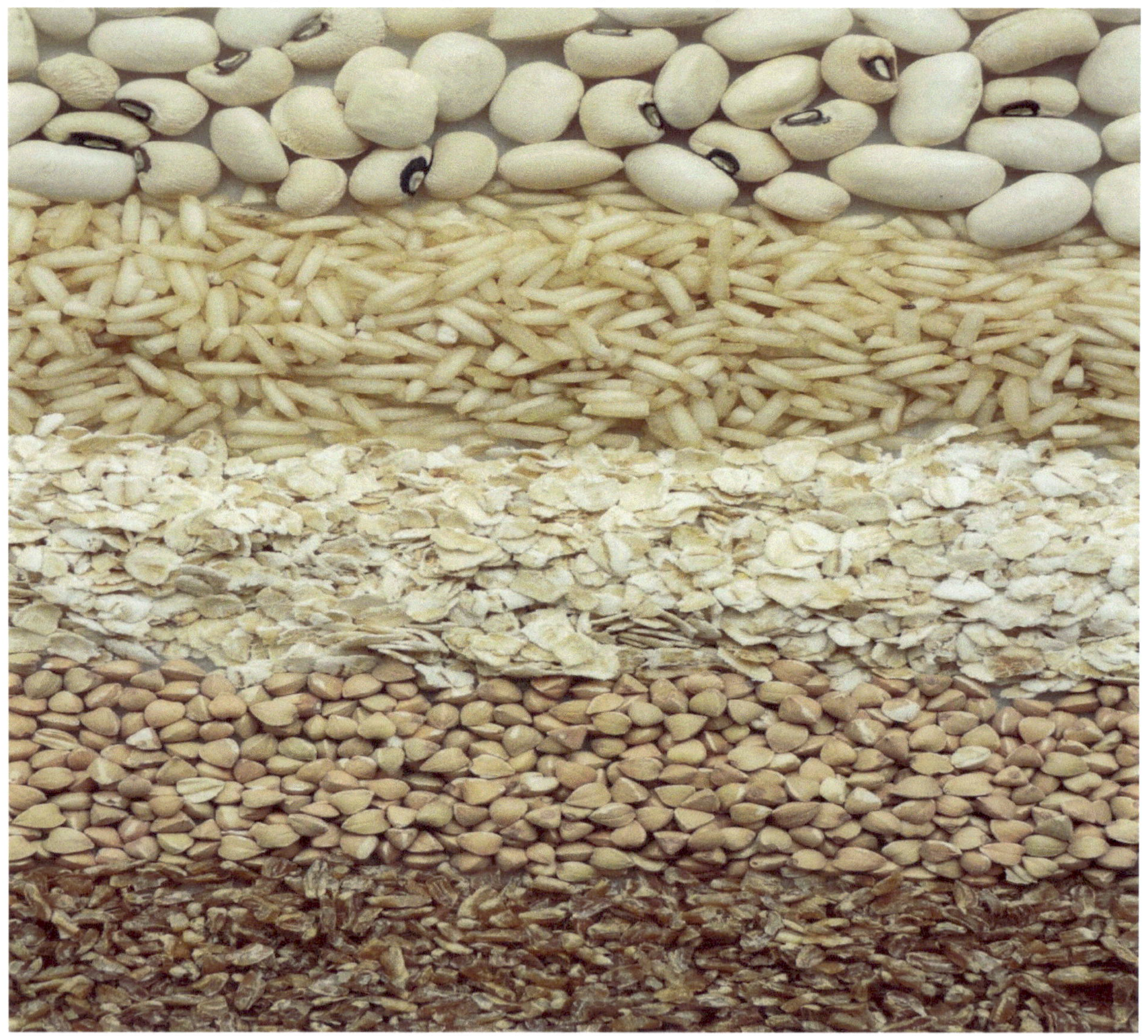

Beans are probably the best wellspring of plant protein. Peas, beans, and chickpeas are aggregately known as vegetables. Most normal beans have 215 calories for each cooked cup (lima beans go up to 260). They have the most protein with the most un-fat of any food, and they're high in potassium yet low in sodium.

Plant protein is deficient, which implies that you have to add something to make it complete. Consolidate beans with an entire grain – rice, grain, wheat, corn – to give the amino acids important to frame a total protein. At that point, you get a similar top-quality protein as in meat with simply a small amount of the fat.

Studies at the University of Kentucky and in the Netherlands show that eating beans routinely can bring down cholesterol levels.

The most well-known protest about beans is that they cause gas. Here's how to contain that issue, as per the U.S. Branch of Horticulture (USDA): Before cooking, flush the beans and eliminate unfamiliar particles, place in a pot and cover with bubbling water, drench for four hours or more, eliminate any beans that buoy to the top, at that point cook the beans in new water.

Berries

https://18c10dji3polfumgzz4x6xcj0n.hop.clickbank.net/

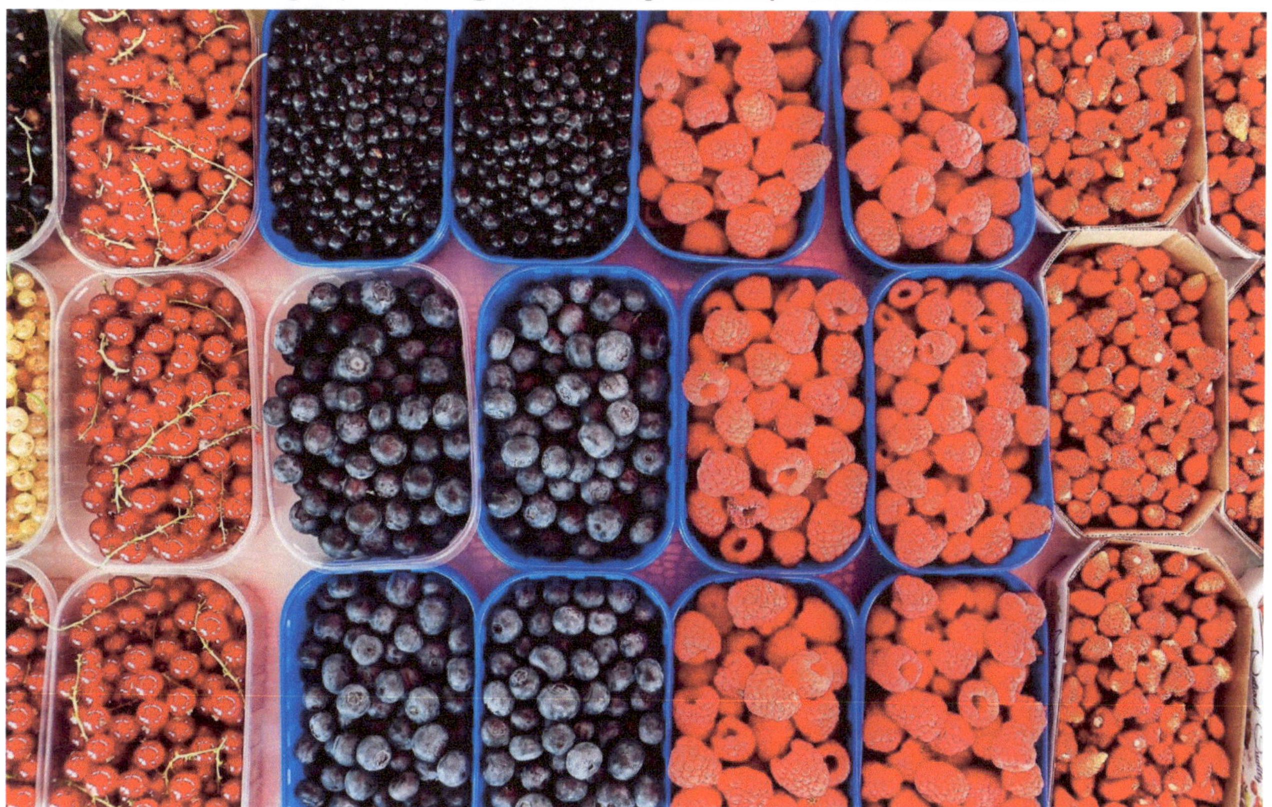

This is the ideal weight reduction food. Berries have regular fructose sugar that fulfills your yearning for desserts and enough fiber so you assimilate fewer calories that you eat. English specialists found that the high substance of insoluble fiber in natural products, vegetables, and entire grains diminishes the ingestion of calories from nourishments enough to advance with misfortune without hampering sustenance.

Berries are an incredible wellspring of potassium that can help you in circulatory strain control. Blackberries have 74 calories for each cup, blueberries 81, raspberries 60, and strawberries 45. So utilize your creative mind and appreciate your preferred berry.

Broccoli

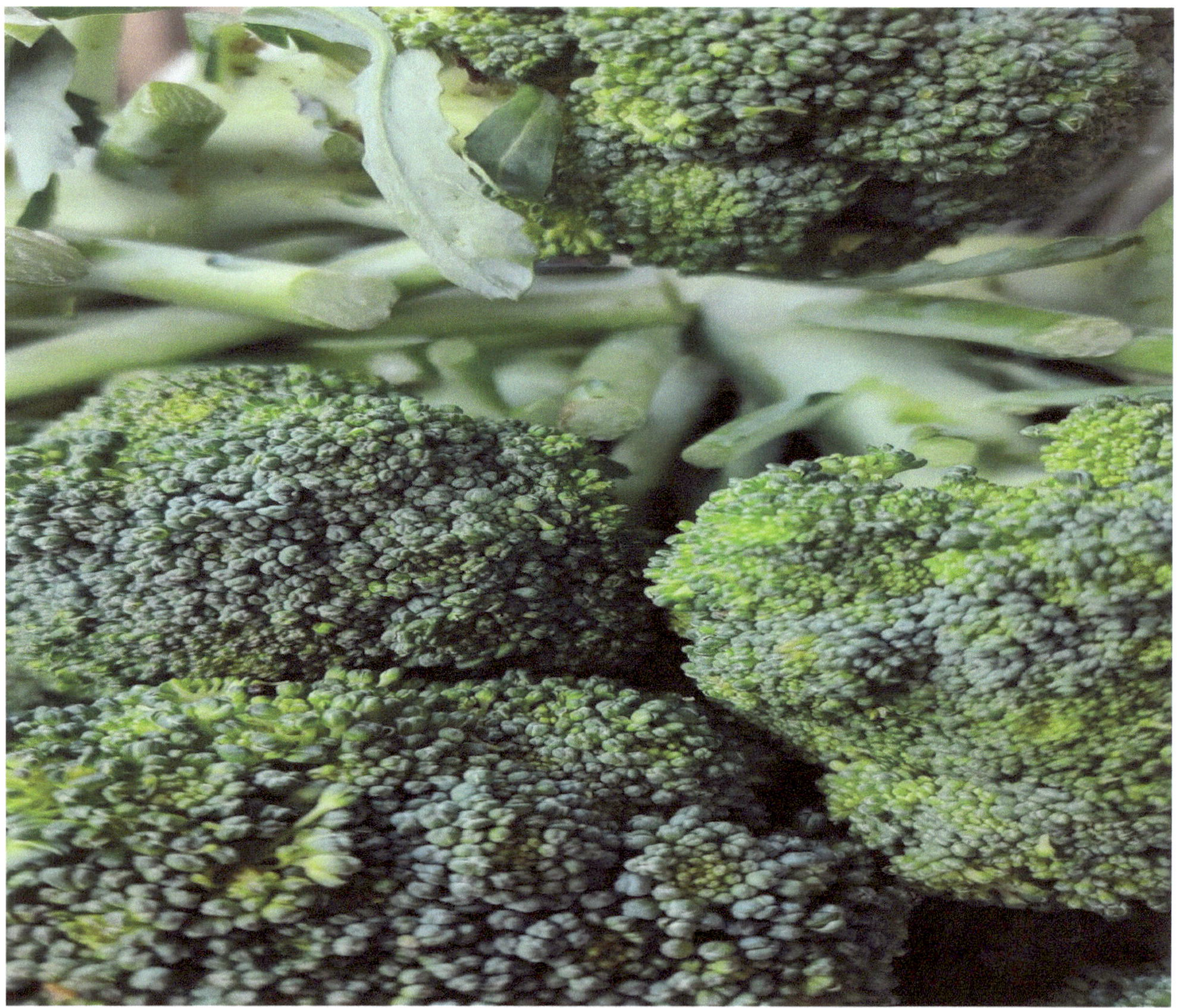

Broccoli is America's number one vegetable, as per an ongoing survey. No big surprise. A cup of cooked broccoli has a simple 44 calories. It conveys a stunning dietary payload and is viewed as the main disease battling vegetable. It has no fat, heaps of fiber, malignancy battling synthetics called indoles, carotene, multiple times the RDA of nutrient C and calcium.

At the point when you're purchasing broccoli, focus on the shading. The minuscule florets should be rich green and free of yellowing. Stems should be firm.

`
Buckwheat
https://be824hen4nnrf7m8t9qdwh6w2v.hop.clickbank.net/

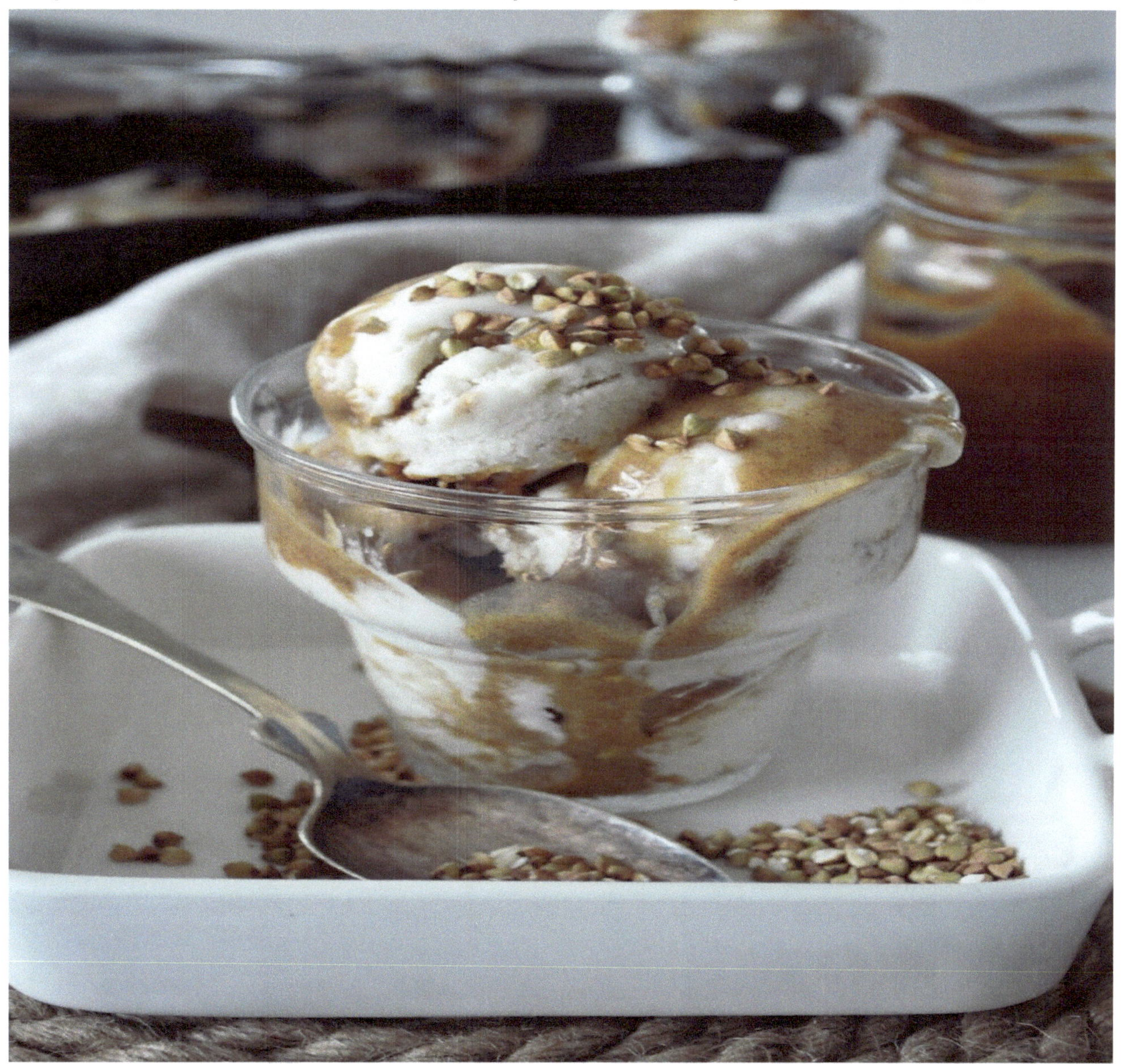

It's extraordinary for hotcakes, pieces of bread, oats, soups, or alone as a grain dish regularly called kasha. It has 155 calories for every cooked cup. Examination at the All India Organization of Clinical Sciences shows eating less including buckwheat leads to magnificent glucose guidelines, protection from diabetes, and brings down cholesterol levels. You cook buckwheat a similar way you would rice or grain. Heat a few cups of water to the point of boiling, add the grain, cover the container, turn down the warmth, and stew for 20 minutes or until the water is assimilated.

Cabbage

https://be824hen4nnrf7m8t9qdwh6w2v.hop.clickbank.net/

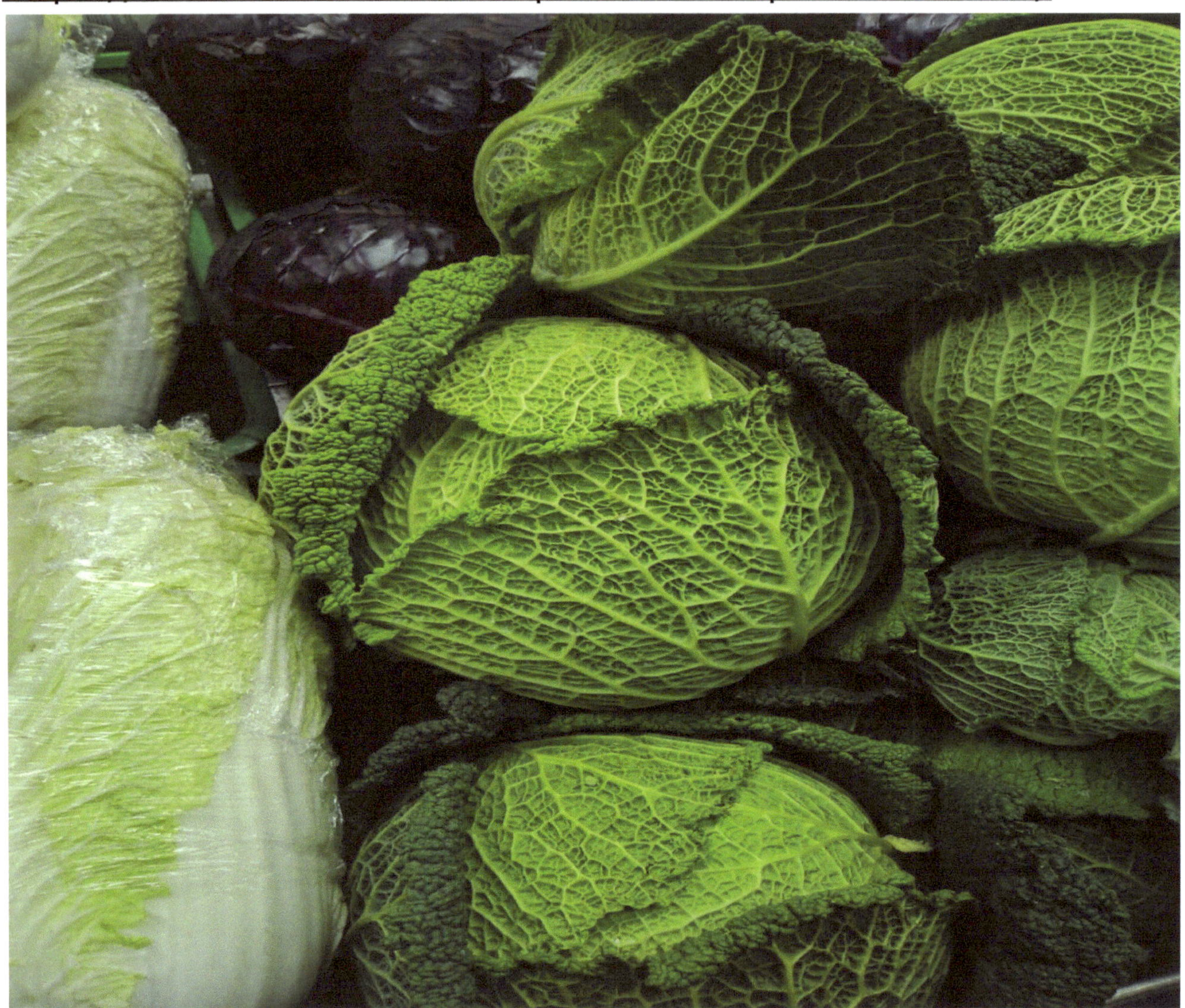

This Eastern European staple is a true wonder food. There are only 33 calories in a cup of cooked shredded cabbage, and it retains all its nutritional goodness no matter how long you cook it. Eating cabbage raw (18 calories per shredded cup), cooked, as sauerkraut (27 calories per drained cup) or coleslaw (calories depend on the dressing) only once a week is enough to protect against colon cancer. And it may be a longevity-enhancing food. Surveys in the United States, Greece, and Japan show that people who eat a lot of it have the least colon cancer and the lowest death rates overall.

Carrots

https://be824hen4nnrf7m8t9qdwh6w2v.hop.clickbank.net/

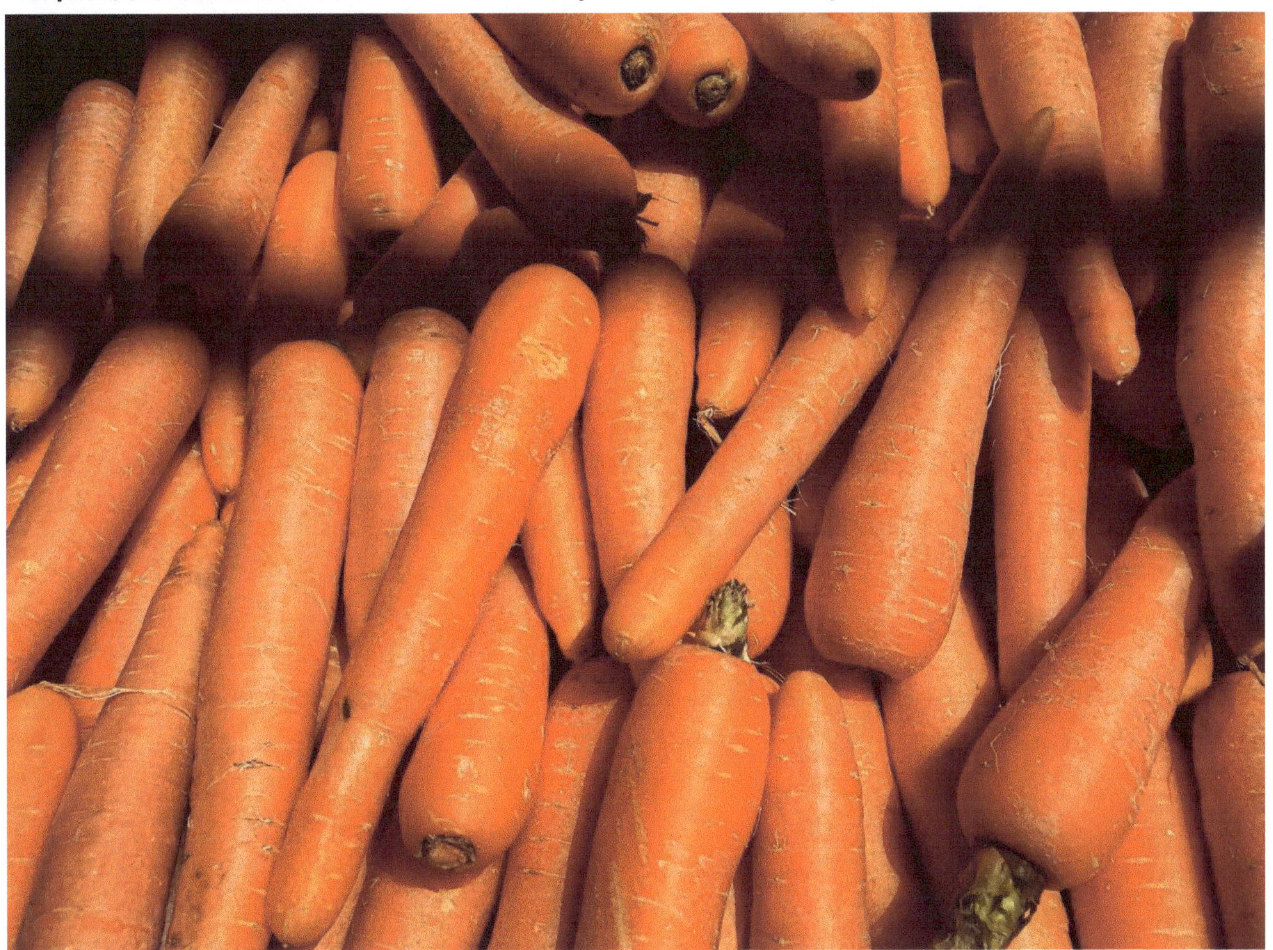

What list of health-promoting, fat-fighting foods would be complete without Bugs Bunny's favorite? A medium-sized carrot carries about 55 calories and is a nutritional powerhouse. The orange color comes from beta carotene, a powerful cancer-preventing nutrient (provitamin A).

Chop and toss them with pasta, grate them into rice or add them to a stir-fry. Combine them with parsnips, oranges, raisins, lemon juice, chicken, potatoes, broccoli, or lamb to create flavorful dishes. Spice them with tarragon, dill, cinnamon, or nutmeg. Add finely chopped carrots to soups and spaghetti sauce – they impart a natural sweetness without adding sugar.

Chicken

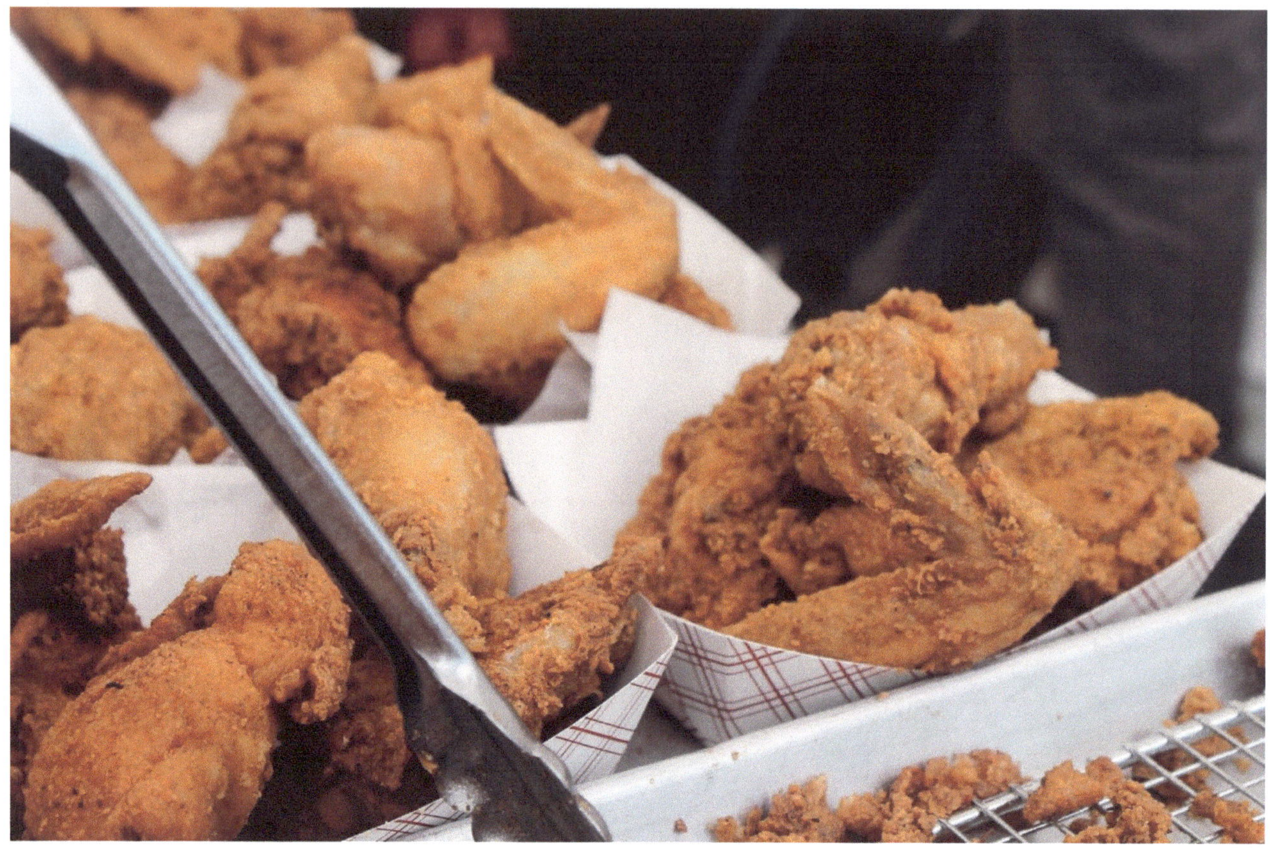

White meat contains 245 calories per four ounces serving and dark meat, 285. It's an excellent source of protein, iron, niacin, and zinc. Skinned chicken is healthiest, but most experts recommend waiting until after cooking to remove it because the skin keeps the meat moist during cooking.

<u>Corn</u>

<u>https://be824hen4nnrf7m8t9qdwh6w2v.hop.clickbank.net/</u>

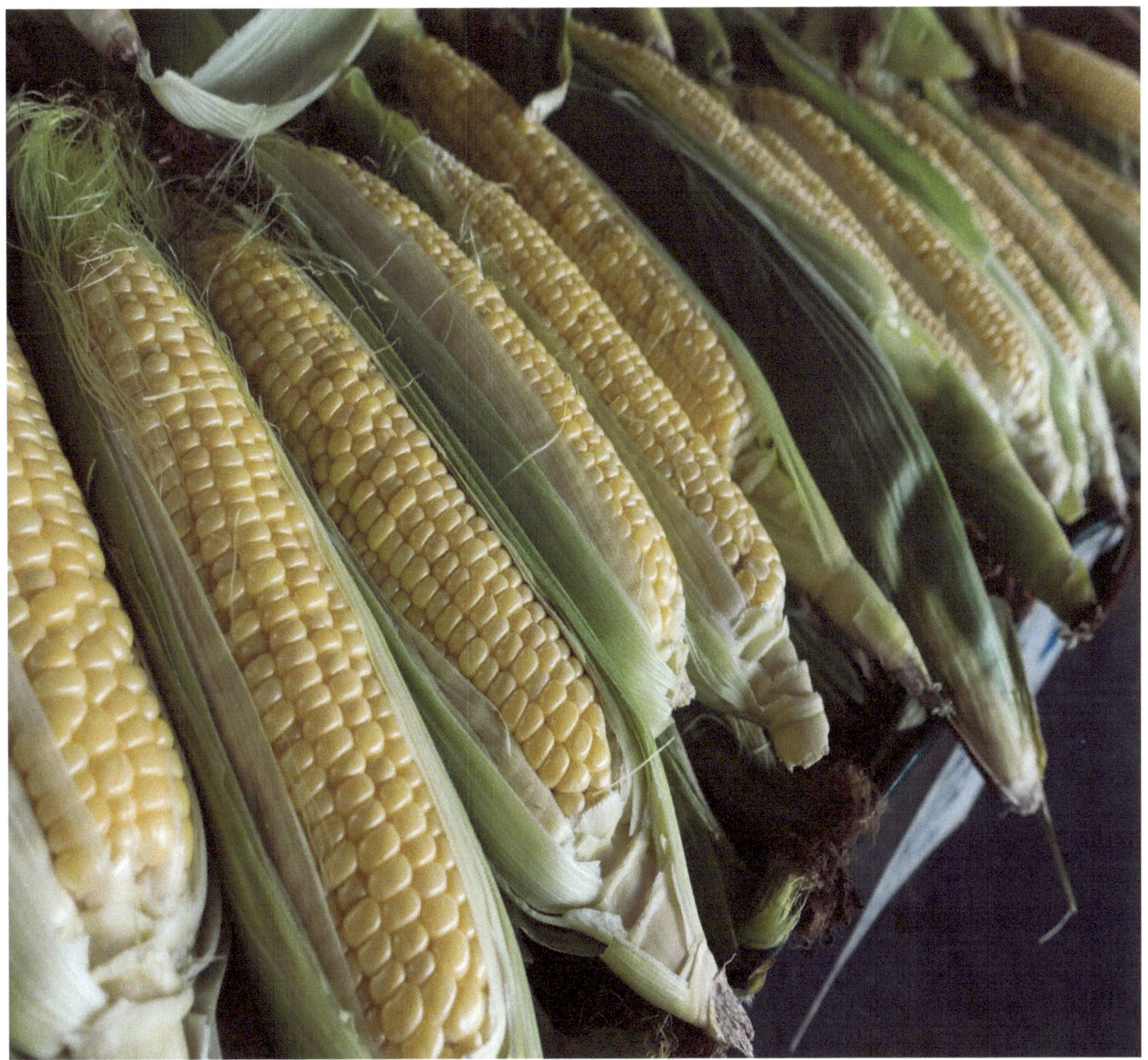

It's a grain – not a vegetable – and is another food that's gotten a bum rap. People think it has little to offer nutritionally and that just isn't so. There are 178 calories in a cup of cooked kernels. It contains good amounts of iron, zinc, and potassium, and the University of Nebraska researchers say it delivers a high-quality protein, too.

The Tarahumara Indians of Mexico eat corn, beans, and hardly anything else. Virgil Brown, M.D., of Mount Sinai School of Medicine in New York, points out that high blood cholesterol and cardiovascular heart disease are almost nonexistent among them.

Cottage Cheese

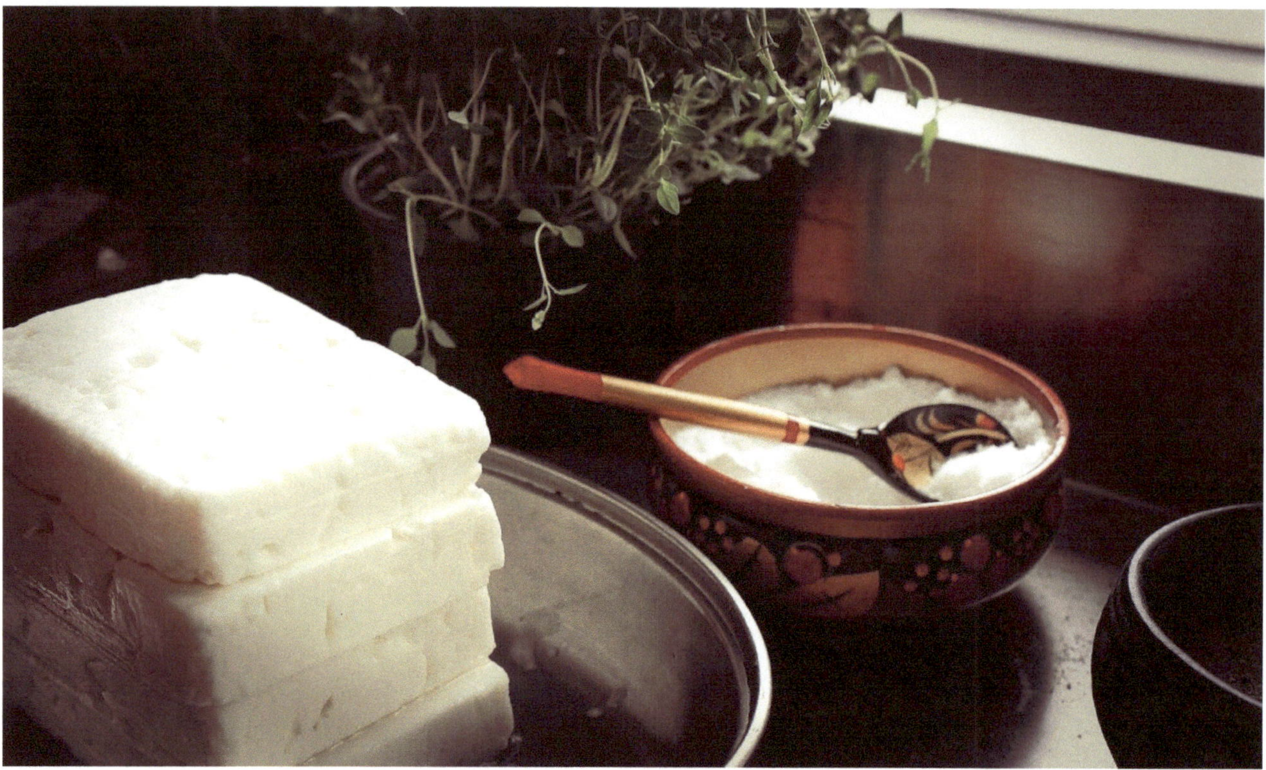

As long as we're talking about losing weight and fat-fighting foods, we had to mention cottage cheese.

Low-fat (2%) cottage cheese has 205 calories per cup and is admirably low in fat while providing respectable amounts of calcium and the B vitamin riboflavin. Season with spices such a dill, or garden fresh vegetables such as scallions and chives for extra zip.

To make it sweeter, add raisins or one of the fruit spreads with no sugar added. You can also use cottage cheese in cooking, baking, fillings, and dips where you would otherwise use sour cream or cream cheese.

Figs

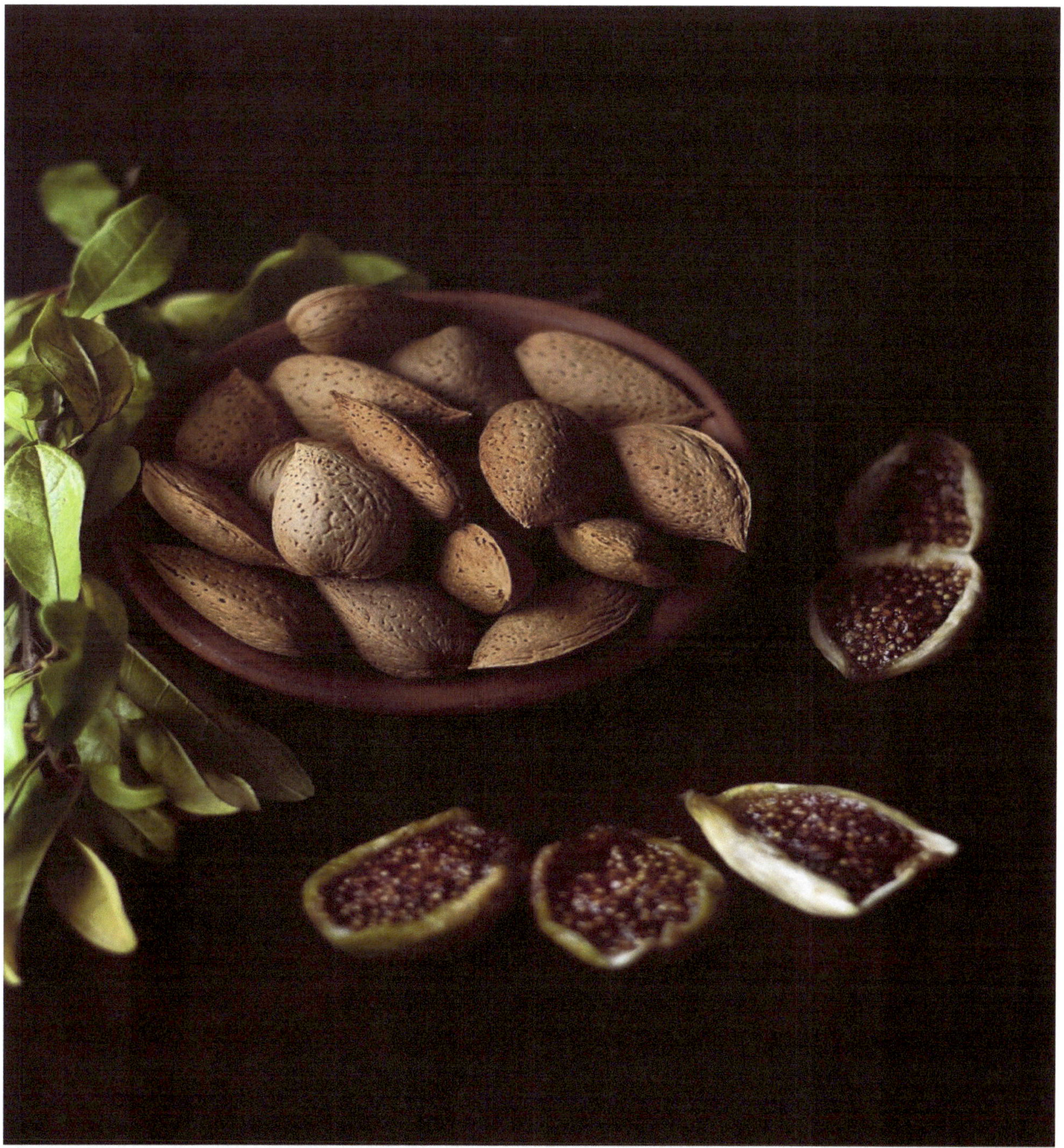

Fiber-rich figs are low in calories at 37 per medium (2.25″ diameter) raw fig and 48 per dried fig. A recent study by the USDA demonstrated that they contribute to a feeling of fullness and prevent overeating. Subjects complained of being asked to eat too much food when fed a diet containing more figs than a similar diet with an identical number of calories.

Serve them with other fruits and cheeses. Or poach them in fruit juice and serve them warm or cold. You can stuff them with mild white cheese or puree them to use as a filling for cookies and low-calorie pastries.

Fish
https://be824hen4nnrf7m8t9qdwh6w2v.hop.clickbank.net/

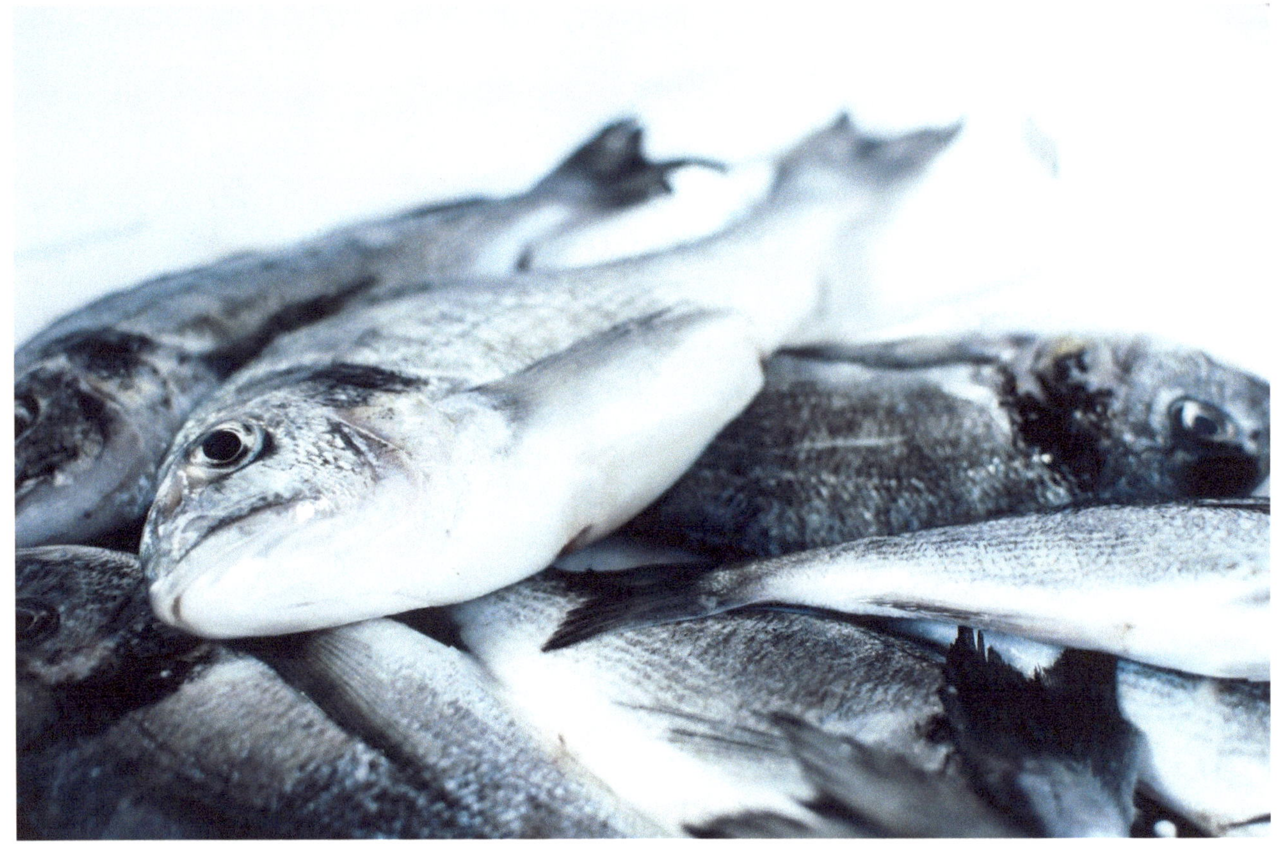

The health benefits of fish are greater than experts imagined – and they've always considered it a healthy food.

The calorie count in the average four-ounce serving of a deep-sea fish runs from a low of 90 calories in abalone to a high of 236 in herring. Water-packed tuna, for example, has 154 calories. It's hard to gain weight eating seafood.

As far back as 1985, articles in the New England Journal of Medicine showed a clear link between eating fish regularly and lower rates of heart disease. The reason is that oils in fish thin the blood, reduce blood pressure, and lower cholesterol.

Dr. Joel Kremer, at Albany Medical College in New York, discovered that daily supplements of fish oil brought dramatic relief to the inflammation and stiff joints of rheumatoid arthritis.

Greens

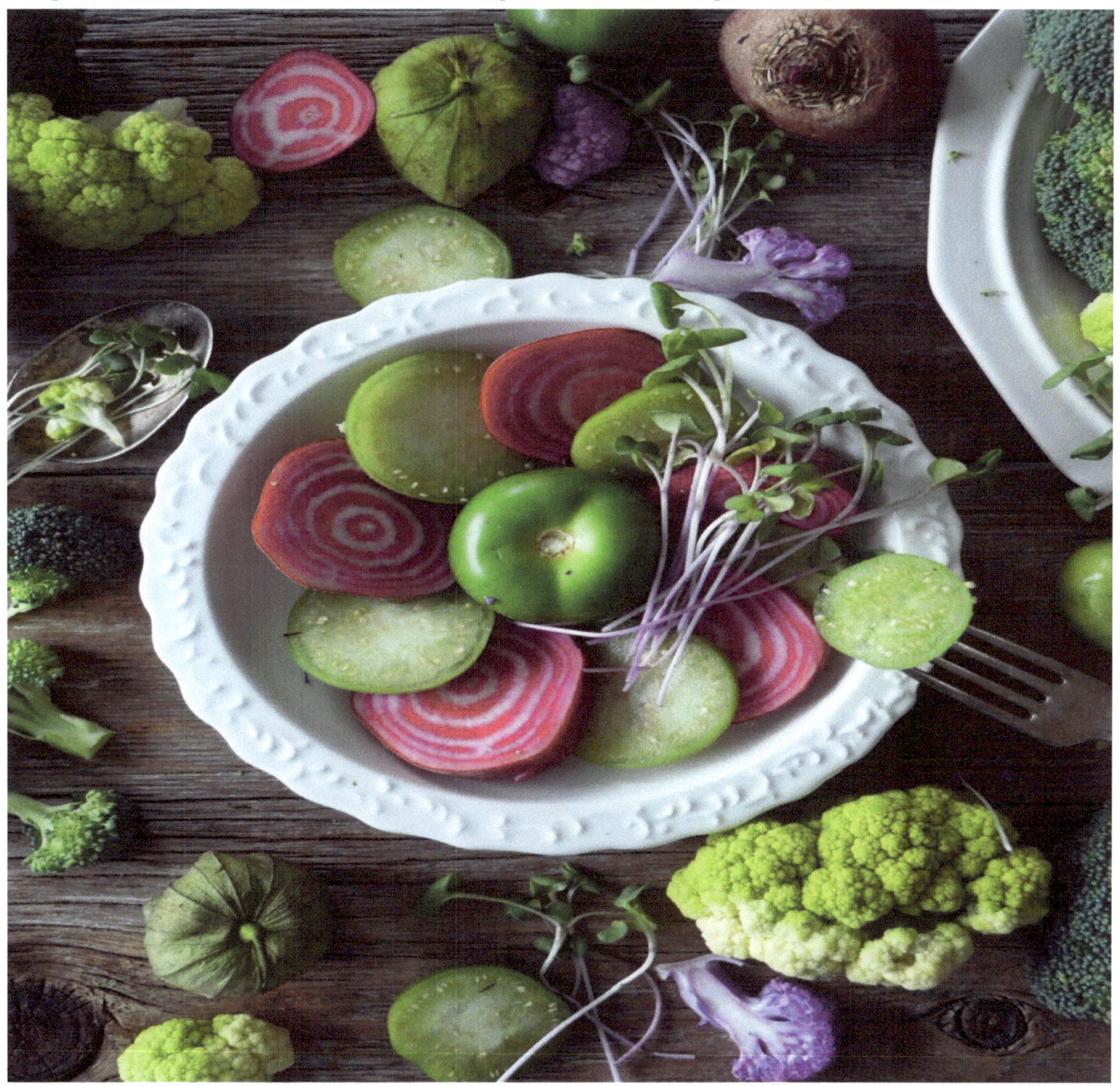

We're talking collard, chicory, beet, kale, mustard, Swiss chard, and turnip greens. They all belong to the same family as spinach, and that's one of the super-stars. No matter how hard you try, you can't load a cup of plain cooked greens with any more than 50 calories.

They're full of fiber, loaded with vitamins A and C and free of fat. You can use them in salads, soups, etc.

www.ingramcontent.com/pod-product-compliance
Lightning Source LLC
Chambersburg PA
CBHW040202240726

48664CB00002B/803